610.73

Key

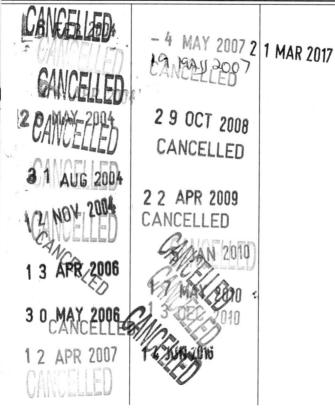

Don Gresswell Ltd., London, N21   Cat. No. 1207   DG 02242/71

Key Nursing Skills

BARBARA A WORKMAN
RGN, MSc, BSc(Hons), RNT, RCNT,
Dip N(Lond)
Senior Lecturer, Middlesex University

CLARE L BENNETT
RGN, MA, BSc(Hons), DipN,
PGCHE
Senior Lecturer, Middlesex University

With contributions from

FRANCES GORDON
PhD, MEd, RN, RNT, RCNT
Principal Lecturer, Middlesex University

NORA COOPER
RGN, BA(Hons), PGCEA
Senior Lecturer, Middlesex University

W
WHURR PUBLISHERS
LONDON AND PHILADELPHIA

© 2003 Whurr Publishers Ltd
First published 2003 by
Whurr Publishers Ltd
19b Compton Terrace, London N1 2UN, England and
325 Chestnut Street, Philadelphia PA19106, USA

Reprinted 2003 (twice)

British Library Cataloguing in Publication Data

A catalogue record for this book is available from the
British Library.

ISBN 1 86156 322 1

Printed and bound in the UK by Athenaeum Press
Limited, Gateshead, Tyne & Wear

Contents

Preface

The authors, who all have wide experience in teaching and practising adult nursing, collaborated to write this book, which evolved from a clinical skills module. It became apparent that students loved learning the introductory nursing skills, but there were few easily accessible texts to support their learning. This book is therefore aimed at nursing students embarking on their nursing education, although some of it will also be suitable for care assistants who are involved in delivering direct nursing care to patients. It may also be useful as a teaching resource for qualified nurses who provide support to learners in the clinical area and those who are returning to practice who need to be clinically updated. The book is not intended to be a substitute for appropriate supervision in clinical practice, and no responsibility can be taken by the writers or publisher for any damage or injury to persons or property.

As the emphasis is on introductory skills there are inevitable omissions of specific procedures. Once the introductory skills have been acquired, new skills can be learnt easily as principles for practice will be transferable to the new situation.

Each chapter focuses on a specific area of care and related skills. Each intervention is presented within a 'Nursing problem' that states the nature of the patient problem and then the goal. The currently available evidence base is outlined and related to the problem before the procedure is explained in simple steps. Experienced nurses' tips have been integrated into the procedures, so alerting the learner to anticipate individual patients' needs or anxieties, or to improve upon their own performance. Each chapter concludes with key texts to supplement the procedural steps with more theory. However, the book is not a substitute for detailed study of broader nursing texts and we must emphasize that although there is a lot of detail in some procedures, knowledge and understanding of the full nursing curriculum should be further pursued.

Where applicable, specific terms have been defined to aid learners in developing their own vocabulary of specialist words, and to remind them that nursing jargon is also incomprehensible to patients. Another language issue is gender: both nurses and patients can be either male or female. However, to avoid the constant repetition of phrases such as *he or she* throughout this book nurses are generally referred to by using *she* or *her*, and patients by using *he* or *him*, and so on, except where a specific patient is being discussed. This does not imply any assumptions by the authors about typical nurses or patients, and is merely intended to simplify the text.

Section I introduces a structured approach to aid patient assessment. Although this is not an actual 'procedure', it is one that is done so automatically by experienced nurses that the knowledge and observation skills used are often not made explicit. We have tried to articulate many of these skills. We know from our contact with students that the opportunity to work with experienced nurses is highly valued and very beneficial: it offers the opportunity to learn more than just fundamental care because it provides a rich source of nursing knowledge and skill. Development of such skills in assessment is vital when planning, implementing and evaluating care.

Section II addresses nursing skills that are fundamental to a patient's wellbeing, recovery or comfort. These are skills that are often delegated to students or care assistants because they apparently do not require much technical knowledge. The delivery of safe and effective care, using evidence-based principles, is as essential here as more technical care. It requires knowledge and theoretical understanding, and application of principles such as infection control and patient comfort. These are the kind of skills that make a patient feel really 'well nursed' – or not, as the case may be – and are central to providing a caring environment for recovery and comfort.

Section III details technical skills that student nurses are frequently involved in, and outlines more detailed knowledge and procedures for effective nursing practice. Where appropriate the interventions are cross-referenced between chapters. For example, methods of respiratory medication are included in Chapter 8 on respiratory care, but the principles of drug administration are in Chapter 6. The final chapter, on principles of pre- and post-operative care, draws on other interventions from throughout the book, and provides a useful summary of their application.

The report *Fitness for Practice* (UKCC 1999) identified that nursing skills were deficient in the diploma preparation for nursing. It is hoped that the nursing interventions described here will contribute to rectifying this deficiency and provide a solid basis for acquiring essential nursing skills.

We hope that this book will be useful and informative, and that it will contribute to the delivery of high quality nursing care.

Barbara Workman
Clare Bennett
August 2002

Acknowledgements

We thank our students for giving us the incentive and initial enthusiasm to write this book, and our colleagues, especially Sheila Quinn and Brian Anthony, for providing support and encouragement. Particular thanks are due to Middlesex University for providing sabbatical leave for Barbara to collate and edit the contents. Thanks also to our illustrators, Bettina Bennett and Julia Twinam, and to the Royal Free Hospital Trust for use of their neurological observation chart.

Last but not least, our grateful thanks to our respective long-suffering husbands, and Louise and Ralph, who provided support and encouragement throughout the creative process.

Assessment procedures

CHAPTER 1

Beginning the assessment process

Barbara Workman and Nora Cooper

Aims and learning outcomes

This chapter aims to introduce you to the fundamental skills and knowledge needed to assess a patient's needs for care. By the end of the chapter you should be able to:

- explain why assessment is important
- understand how assessment informs the planning of care
- use a structured approach to gain a patient history and interpret findings
- describe how discharge is planned starting from admission.

Assessment procedures

It is important to appreciate that assessment is fundamental to all procedures that a patient may undergo. It does not happen just once but is an ongoing process repeated at regular intervals depending on the patient's condition. The most usual time for a thorough assessment to occur is when a patient is admitted to acute or continuing care, but there may be other times when further detailed assessment is necessary.

Assessing a patient involves both formal and informal assessment. Formal assessment includes the gathering of objective information about the patient's condition by interviewing him or her and obtaining answers to questions. Informal assessment includes the things that you notice about a patient while you are talking to them, and may include physical signs and subjective information such as their mood or behaviour. The structure of these assessments will be discussed in more detail in this chapter. Assessment of physical vital signs is also undertaken and these are described more fully in Chapter 2. An effective assessment will ensure that a patient receives all the nursing care that is required, and will provide a baseline from which progress can be measured. To ensure that nursing care is planned and delivered effectively a structured approach called the 'nursing process' is used.

The 'nursing process' is a planned, problem-solving approach to meeting a patient's health care and nursing needs (Lippincott 2000). It is a systematic sequence of events in which the first stage is to assess a patient's needs by the collection of objective and subjective information. The next stage is interpretation of this information, which results in the identification of actual or potential problems that the patient is experiencing. This can be called making a nursing diagnosis (Lippincott 2000). Nursing goals to alleviate or prevent these problems can then be determined and problems prioritized so that the patient's immediate nursing care needs are met. These goals are used to plan the direction and type of nursing interventions required. They should be patient-focused, and SMART:

Specific

Measurable

Achievable

Realistic

Timebound

For example, a patient may state his problem as being extreme breathlessness at rest. A short-term goal may be that his respiration rate will be 25–28 breaths per minute within four hours. This would allow time for medication and nursing measures to take effect. This goal statement fulfils the SMART requirements, and would be followed by specific nursing interventions that would contribute to achieving the goal (see Chapter 8). There are examples of problems and goals throughout this book, together with nursing interventions to meet the goals.

When nursing interventions have been implemented the results should be evaluated. Evaluation provides the opportunity to see how the patient responded to the nursing interventions and the extent to which the goals have been achieved (Lippincott 2000). As a result of evaluation it may be necessary to change goals, as previous problems may no longer exist and new ones may become apparent. If goals are not achieved then the problem should be reconsidered and the goals and interventions revised.

The whole sequence of the nursing process, therefore, is:

assessment – collection of objective and subjective information

nursing diagnosis – identification of potential or actual health problems

planning – plan of care interventions to resolve or address identified problems

implementation – delivery of nursing interventions

evaluation – appraisal of effectiveness of nursing interventions and degree of progress towards resolving the problem.

While the nursing process provides a framework in which to deliver nursing care, a nursing model provides a structure in which care is delivered. It considers the role of the nurse, the needs of the patient and the intended aims of the care as it is delivered. A nursing model is compiled of beliefs and values about people, society, the environment, health and nursing, and encompasses the social, physical and psychological aspects of health in each of these areas (Pearson et al. 1996). Ideally, the nursing model should be chosen to respond to individual patients' needs (Roper et al. 1998). For example, a patient requiring a period of rehabilitation following a road traffic accident will benefit from a model that encourages gradual return to independence rather than depending on health care professionals. Alternatively, a patient with a terminal disease may become steadily more dependent on health care professionals to meet his physical care needs, and the focus of care would be on providing comfort and symptom relief and to make the most of his remaining time. Whatever nursing model is chosen in your clinical area, it is intended to enhance nursing care delivery by being explicit about the nature and purpose of that care, and to provide a structure for recording and documenting observations and actions, thus promoting continuity of care (Iyer and Camp 1999).

When skilled practitioners are observed making an assessment it is often difficult to see how they gained all their information, as they make a complicated process appear simple. It may look more like an informal conversation between the patient and nurse than a structured assessment. But the experience of interacting with patients and the ability to identify essential information guides the conversation and aids collection of information. When first admitting a patient into your care there are certain specific assessment activities that will be undertaken, and as these are completed they gather the required information. These activities are: first impressions, assessment interview, focused assessment and physical assessment.

First impressions

Part of your assessment will include some of the first impressions that you notice about the patient. As you become more experienced you will develop these observation skills. While you are settling the patient into the ward you will already be observing him. Springhouse (2002) offers a mnemonic checklist – SOME TEAMS – to help guide you through key patient observations:

Symmetry:
Are his face and body symmetrical? Are there any swellings of joints or body parts?

Old:
Does he look his age? If not, can you see why?

Mental acuity:
Is he alert, confused, agitated, inattentive or responding inappropriately? Is his mood depressed, happy or lethargic?

Expression:
Does he appear ill, in pain, anxious or distressed?

Trunk:
Is he lean, wasted, stocky, obese or barrel-chested?

Extremities:
Does he have joint abnormalities, or oedema? Does he have warm or cold hands and feet? Is his skin pale, well perfused or with a bluish (cyanotic) tinge?

Appearance:

Is he clean, well kept and appropriately dressed? Has he inadequate or excessive clothing on for the time of year? Is his skin in good condition or are there signs of rashes, bruising, dry skin or infestation?

Movement:

Are his posture, gait and coordination normal? Can he manipulate buttons and zips with his fingers, or reach to take off his shoes?

Speech:

Is his speech relaxed, clear, strong, understandable and appropriate? Does he sound anxious, stressed, slurred or rambling?

These initial informal observations can give subtle clues about a patient's health, and are useful to reflect upon later if you think there are changes in the patient's condition, but are unable to pinpoint exactly what those changes might be.

Assessment interview

Introductions

When you first meet the patient, introduce yourself and address him respectfully using his proper title. This allows him to choose what he would like to be called during his stay. If he is an inpatient, introduce him to the other patients in his room and show him around the clinical area so that he knows where the toilets and bath or shower rooms are, and where to find the telephone or day room. It is often a patient's first experience of health care and he may be nervous. It is worth taking time to put him at ease and explain who will be caring for him from the multi-disciplinary team and how to distinguish between the uniforms of the varying staff he is likely to meet. If English is not his first language, you may find out at this stage that there is a language barrier, so before you progress to the interview, see if you can find an interpreter.

TIP! If a patient needs an interpreter, family members may be keen to help, but some private details of a patient's condition may not be suitable for a family member, particularly a child, to interpret. For example, a woman may not find it easy to talk about period irregularities if her son is the family translator; it may be more appropriate to use official interpreters.

Preparing to interview

Before interviewing the patient it is important to prepare yourself and the patient for the assessment interview. Explain that you need to gather some information and ensure that it is a convenient time to interview him. The patient may like to visit the toilet, change his position, receive some pain relief, or say goodbye to relatives first. You will need to gather the key biographical details from the medical notes so that you can verify details of such information as date of birth, address and contact numbers of the next of kin.

TIP! If a relative is the main carer it may be useful to include them in some of the interview, or to check some details with them separately. However, the patient must know that all information that he gives you will be regarded as confidential and only passed onto other health care professionals if necessary. In some circumstances it may be particularly important that both the carer and the patient are able to express their real feelings and anxieties out of the hearing of the other. This should be handled sensitively and may not happen at initial assessment.

Interview atmosphere

Provide a comfortable and quiet place in which to conduct the interview if possible, and ensure that you are not so close to the patient that you invade his personal space, but not so far away that you have to shout. Ensure that the patient can see you and that you are not positioned with the light behind you. Aim for a calm, unhurried and non-judgemental atmosphere. By giving the patient time and attention he is more likely to relax and open up and impart all the information that you need. If you show disapproval, disgust or impatience this may block communication (Bates and Hoekelman 2000), so you need to develop a professional demeanour that does not make a patient feel guilty or vulnerable about some aspects of his lifestyle – for example, his alcohol or tobacco consumption.

Effective communication

Be aware that some medical jargon may prevent the patient from understanding the questions you are asking, so use layman's language and terms. Encourage the patient as he talks by nodding your head and saying things like 'Go on'. Help him to tell his own story by asking questions, such as 'Can you tell me when this problem started?'.

Nonverbal communication can tell you about the person too. Listen carefully, and watch for body language signals. If a person is uncomfortable about an aspect of your questions he may not make eye contact. Some cultures, however, may consider eye contact as disrespectful or aggressive and may not meet your eyes at all during the interview (Springhouse 2002). It is important to check that you have understood the signals correctly. For example, if a patient is holding himself as if in pain, you could ask a question such as 'You look very uncomfortable just now, can you tell me how you are feeling?' This gives the opportunity to talk about any pain he may be feeling or any worries he may have. Outbursts of anger, aggression, tears or rudeness are types of nonverbal behaviour that communicate feelings such as anxiety, insecurity and fear.

TIP! Some patients have to tell their stories so many times that it exhausts them, so start your assessment with the really important things first, especially for emergency admissions. You can fill in the gaps from the following: medical records, letters from other health professionals, communications from ambulance staff, accident and emergency records or friends and relatives.

There are a wide variety of communication skills that can be used when interviewing. Closed questions are used to get one- or two-word answers, and are useful for confirming specific information such as personal address details. Open questions provide the opportunity to express feelings and ideas, and for the patient to recount his experience. Bates and Hoekelman (2000) identify other communication strategies to use to elicit information:

Facilitation:
This encourages the patient to continue his story. You may use an attentive position such as leaning forward and nodding, or a listening silence while the patient gathers his thoughts.

Reflection:
Repeating back to the patient the words that he has just said can help him to gather his thoughts and elaborate further.

Confirmation:

This makes sure you are both on the right track and clears any misconceptions.

Clarification:

If the patient is a bit vague or ambiguous you can ask him to explain some more.

Ask about feelings:

You can ask the patient what he felt about a situation or events as this may allow him to express anxiety, anger or fear.

Summarizing:

This is restating the information that has been given to you to draw it together.

Conclusion:

This signals the end of the interview but offers the patient the opportunity to tell you something he may like to add.

Structure of assessment interview

Bates and Hoekelman (2000) outline the structure of the assessment interview as covering the following areas:

- biographical data
- reason for admission
- past medical history
- family history
- the ability to meet daily living activities
- any psychosocial factors that may affect health
- physical assessment of vital signs (see Chapter 2).

Additional, more focused assessment may be undertaken on any particular aspects of daily living such as nutrition (Chapter 9), breathing (Chapter 8), continence (Chapter 10) or other specific areas depending on the patient's needs and identified problems.

Recording information

Most assessment forms have specific areas that require completion in writing, and this may follow the structure of the chosen nursing model.

Without experience you may be heavily reliant on paper and worrying about the next question to be asked, and not able to watch for clues from the patient about their real feelings. You may find it helpful to have some notepaper with you to take down some key points that you can then record clearly in the correct order on the local documentation later. Make sure you explain to the patient that you want to record details accurately. Jot down key phrases and dates rather than the full story, especially when discussing complex problems. There may be some moments in the interview when it is more appropriate to be listening rather than writing, particularly if the patient is talking about sensitive or distressing issues (Bates and Hoekelman 2000).

Biographical data

Start by checking biographical details. This should include the patient's full name, address, telephone number, date of birth, age, marital status and religion. A contact number of someone who can be called in an emergency should be included and this may be a next of kin or, if they live some distance away, it may be a partner or spouse. It is usual to find out who could be contacted at night, especially if the partner or spouse is elderly and infirm. Patients may be concerned about the implications of having to call someone in an emergency, and so it is wise to explain that it is usual practice to ensure all contact details are current and an emergency number is very rarely needed.

Enquiring as to whether the patient practises his stated religion provides an opportunity for him to express whether he will want to follow particular religious observances, such as attending a service or saying prayers at particular times. There may be particular cultural practices that he would wish to follow during illness, and facilities should be made available for him to do so where possible. Further information about cultural awareness can be followed up in the recommended further reading texts.

Reason for admission

Use the patient's own words to explain his reason for admission to care. To find out more use the PQRST framework (Springhouse 2002) to direct your questions:

P – provocative or palliative. What helps or worsens the symptoms? Do certain situations such as stress or particular physical positions make a difference?

Q – quality or quantity. What does the symptom look, feel or sound like? Is he experiencing it during the interview? How does it affect his normal activities?

R – region or radiation. Where in the body does the symptom occur? Is anywhere else affected by it?

S – severity. How severe is this symptom on a range of 1 to 10 (10 being most severe)? Is it getting better, worse or staying the same?

T – timing. When did it begin? Did it start gradually or suddenly? How frequently does it happen? How long does it last?

Past medical history

In the UK these key details are recorded in the medical notes, but it is important for nursing staff to find out if there are any allergies to drugs, elastoplast, perfumes or other substances. Previous operations and admissions are summarized so that it is understood as to where this latest event fits into the patient's health experience and how it may influence his reaction to current care.

Find out about current medication: whether it has been prescribed by a doctor, advised by a pharmacist, or if the patient has been dosing himself. For example, this may indicate the degree of discomfort that a patient has been experiencing, if the prescribed pain relief has been ineffective and the patient has been supplementing it with medicines from over the counter without realizing the implications of increasing the dose.

Family history

It is usual to find out whether any diseases such as coronary heart disease, some types of cancer or blood disorders, high blood pressure or diabetes are prevalent in the family.

The ability to meet daily living activities

This part of the assessment will highlight if there are any areas that need a focused assessment. Nursing models as outlined by Pearson et al. (1996) may be used to identify deficits in the ability to meet daily living activities. Specific areas of consideration include the following.

Nutrition

Has the reason for admission affected the patient's appetite? Is he able to shop and cook? Are there any special dietary requirements such as diabetes or religious preferences? See Chapter 9 for more details on nutritional assessment.

TIP! **Ensure the patient is able to complete his menu so that his likes and dislikes are noted. If he requires a special diet, kosher or vegetarian meal make sure it is ordered or he may be presented with a 'spare' meal that does not meet his particular requirements.**

Elimination

What are the patient's normal elimination patterns and have they changed recently? If constipation is a problem what are the normal measures that the patient uses to relieve it? Is urinary frequency or incontinence a problem? More detailed assessment questions can be found in Chapter 10.

Mobility

This includes all types of body movement: walking, moving in bed, and manual dexterity. The amount of assistance required to keep the patient mobile should be considered, and special equipment may be required. For example, following assessment of mobility you may decide that the patient will benefit from using a monkey pole to aid moving in bed, or a walking aid when going to the toilet. It may be appropriate to refer the patient to the physiotherapist for a fuller assessment. If a patient cannot move well they may be at risk of complications of bed-rest (see Chapter 5).

Senses

This should consider sight, hearing, smell, touch and taste. Consideration should be given to whether the patient has hearing difficulties that require a hearing aid, or if he needs to lip-read or use sign language. Problems with sight include the need to wear glasses, and if so what sort: long or short sight; the presence of glaucoma, or tunnel vision. Patients with certain neurological conditions may find their smell or taste senses are temporarily or permanently altered.

Sleep

The patient may have had his sleep and rest disturbed by his current problems so it is important to find out his normal sleep patterns. He may have special night-time rituals such as taking a hot or alcoholic drink, or medication, before bedtime. His sleep may be disturbed due to urinary frequency, or because he cannot assume a particular position in which to sleep because of his illness. For example, if he is breathless, he may not be able to lie down comfortably but finds it difficult sleeping sitting up.

Occupation

A patient's occupation may affect his current problem, and may be a contributory factor, even if he is no longer in paid employment. Work may give a patient a reason to recover from illness or assist in his reha-bilitation. If a person is unemployed or has been made redundant, that will affect his economic status and quite possibly his mental health. A person's illness may also have an impact upon the type of work they are able to pursue, so this information may be pertinent to preparing for discharge.

Use of tobacco, alcohol and other drugs

Find out how many cigarettes or how much tobacco he smokes, or if he has given up. The amount of alcohol that the patient normally con-sumes is also important, and if you are able to ask if he consumes any illicit or recreational drugs this is useful information too. For example, a patient suffering from multiple sclerosis may take cannabis for pain relief and may be quite ready to admit regular usage. However, a person involved in a road traffic accident may be less open about drug or alcohol use. Usual medications – including the contraceptive pill or hormone replacement therapy – need to be recorded too.

TIP! **Because you are in the role of a health professional, the patient may be reluctant to be honest about how much alco-hol, tobacco or illegal drugs he consumes, especially if he thinks there might be a problem with them, or if he feels you** are likely to be judgemental. Don't suggest he needs to start a smoking cessation programme at once, but try to get an honest estimate of how many he smokes a day. For example, rather than saying 'Do you smoke one or two packs a day?', ask him how many packs he buys at a time and how long that will last him.

Psychosocial factors that may affect health

Information about a patient's occupation will have already given some indication of financial status. Ask about accommodation: if it is rented or owned by the patient, or if it has central heating or many stairs, this will give some indication of the quality of the accommodation. If the patient states that he doesn't get out much because the lift rarely works this will have implications when planning his discharge, especially concerning his ability to shop or cook.

Recent experiences of bereavement such as divorce, separation or death of a loved one may affect the patient's mood and usual coping mechanisms. If during the interview you discover that the patient has experienced a recent bereavement, it may seem difficult to know what to say, particularly if you are inexperienced. Very often, the patient appreciates the opportunity to talk about the loss, but as his close friends and family may have heard it all before, he may still need to revisit it, so a listening ear is often invaluable.

TIP! It is helpful to find out if the patient has been receiving any kind of support from social or voluntary services prior to admission. This means that if these services need to be recommenced on discharge, the patient will already be known to the service and this will make referral easier. You also need to check if the organization knows that the patient has been admitted, so that resources are not wasted.

Focused assessment

During the interview you may become aware that the patient has a particular problem with, for instance, mobility. You would then need to explore that area in more detail, or refer the patient to an expert such as a member of the multi-disciplinary team.

TIP! **If a patient is referred to an expert health care professional, ask if you can attend that consultation as an observer so that you can extend your knowledge and skills.**

Preparing for discharge

Preparation for discharge has to be started once the initial assessment is complete. Research by Tierney et al. (1994) showed that the majority of patients and carers were not consulted about discharge arrangements. Two weeks after discharge, half the patients were unable to recall whether they were given any information about their condition or treatment. High proportions of patients were readmitted within three months of discharge, mostly as an emergency. Different health care organizations coordinate discharge planning in a variety of ways. Some institutions employ a discharge-planning nurse, others leave it to the ward team. Essentially, clear lines of communication with the patient, family and all relevant members of the multi-disciplinary team should be started at admission and followed through for a successful discharge.

Driscoll (2000) makes the following recommendations for nursing practice in relation to discharge planning:

● Include the carers of patients in any patient education programmes.
● Be aware that some carers work and therefore have time limitations; consider their health when planning discharges.
● Ensure all members of the multi-disciplinary team are kept well informed of treatment needs.
● Arrange appointments for carers with specific members of the multi-disciplinary team, for example, a dietician for a newly diagnosed diabetic patient.
● Involve patients and carers in decision making when planning the patient's post-discharge care.

After assessment

Once the assessment is complete, and you have conducted the interview and measured appropriate vital signs, you should be able to formulate a care plan with problem statements to ensure the patient gets the care he needs. The problem statement should be patient-centred using language he understands and uses. For example, if the patient states he has difficulty in catching his breath, this describes his problem. Nurses can get caught up in jargon and write that the problem is dyspnoea, rather than use the patient's own words. When the problem has been stated, goal statements are formulated. It is sometimes useful to have achievable and measurable short- and long-term goals, or the patient can get frustrated and feel he has not progressed. The next step is to determine nursing interventions to ensure the goal is achieved, and then to evaluate the effectiveness of the care. There are examples of nursing interventions and how to fulfil them in the following chapters.

TIP! **Many students initially find it difficult to write problem statements related to the patient. You may be inclined to use medical jargon but this does not relate to the patient. Take time to talk to your patient and use his words. Two trained nurses may well differ on wording on problem statements. This does not matter: the important thing is that the patient receives the care he needs.**

Some trusts will have prescribed care plans for particular problems and nursing interventions. These should be used where appropriate as they save time and ensure all relevant care is documented, but patients' individual needs and preferences should be included.

Pre-assessment clinics

In many facilities, patients who are booked for an investigation or surgical procedure may be invited to attend a pre-assessment clinic visit before their admission date. During this visit the nurse has time to prepare the patient for the admission and to explain what will happen during the hospital stay. Routine investigations are carried out: for example, blood tests to identify anaemia, chest x-rays to discover lung problems, or electrocardiograms to detect any heart conditions. If any problems are found these can then be corrected prior to admission.

When the patient is then admitted several days later, they have had time to absorb what is going to happen and will be ready to ask any questions they may have before they undergo surgery. Pre-assessment visits mean that patients are admitted on the morning of their surgery and can spend an extra night at home. Obviously this only works for planned admissions, and is impossible for patients admitted as emergencies. Emergency admissions will not have this opportunity, and the patient may be very frightened if events have been very speedy. The patient will need reassurance that his concerns will be anticipated and his needs met, and he should be given clear explanations of any procedures. It is usual to expect to conduct a full assessment within 24 hours of admission, and to document all prescribed care.

Evaluation

Evaluation determines the success of the nursing care by reviewing all the data collected from assessment and comparing the actual outcome of care with the expected goals (Lippincott 2000). It is like another assessment, but is not as comprehensive as the first assessment. It will focus just on the goals and the extent to which they have been achieved, and the prescribed care may be adjusted if necessary. Dates and actions of evaluation should be noted on the care plan so that progress can be monitored.

This chapter has focused on assessing a patient by using an assessment interview and observing some physical and behavioural characteristics, thereby gathering some subjective and objective data. The following chapter considers assessment of vital signs, which provide significant objective data to evaluate when monitoring a patient's progress.

Further reading

Andrews MM, Boyle JS (1999) Transcultural Concepts in nursing Care, 3rd edn. Philadelphia, PA: Lippincott.

Bates B, Hoekelman RA (2000) Guide to Physical Exam and History Taking, 6th edn. On CD-ROM. Philadelphia, PA: Lippincott, Williams and Wilkins.

Springhouse (2002) Assessment Made Incredibly Easy, 2nd edn. Springhouse, PA: Springhouse Publishing Company.

CHAPTER 2

Observations

Clare Bennett

Aims and learning outcomes

This chapter introduces you to an evidence-based approach to measuring and documenting patients' physical observations. By the end of the chapter you should be able to:

- record the oral, axillary, tympanic and rectal temperature, justifying your choice of method, and discuss normal values
- measure the pulse and apex beat and discuss normal values
- record the blood pressure and interpret the results
- assess the level of consciousness
- perform blood glucose monitoring and interpret the results.

Patient assessment

Assessment of a patient's vital signs includes observations of temperature, pulse, blood pressure, respiratory rate and oxygen saturation, blood glucose levels and level of consciousness. These observations provide an efficient and accurate method of monitoring a patient's condition. They also enable evaluation of response to treatment and early detection of problems.

Observations give vital information about a patient's condition and therefore you have a duty to:

● adhere to the UKCC guidelines concerning documentation (UKCC 1998)
● report any deviations from the norm or baseline to a senior member of staff and/or medical colleague
● ensure that all equipment has been calibrated, is safe and is fully functional
● select appropriate equipment; for example, a correctly sized blood pressure cuff should be used for the patient's upper arm size
● adhere to local infection control policies.

Before observations are taken, the patient should be made comfortable and be encouraged to relax. If the patient has taken even mild exercise he should be allowed to rest for a few minutes. To get an accurate assessment of a patient's condition, pain should be relieved and every effort made to reduce anxiety as these factors may influence the vital signs. Body temperature, posture and certain drugs will also alter a patient's observations.

NURSING PROBLEM 2.1

Patient history: Mr Ellis is a young man and has been admitted to the ward following a head injury. He was knocked unconscious but is now beginning to recover.

Problem: Mr Ellis has an altered level of consciousness.

Goal: To identify promptly any changes in neurological function.

Pulse rate

When the left ventricle of the heart contracts, it forces blood into the aorta and transmits a thrust through the arterial system that can be felt in the peripheral arteries as a pulse.

Assessment of a patient's pulse provides an efficient method of assessing the status of the heart and circulation (Perry and Potter

1998). There are several pulse points on the body, the most common being the radial pulse. The radial artery is located near the radius bone on the thumb side of the wrist. If the radial pulse is inaccessible or if it is irregular, listening to (auscultation of) the pulse at the apex of the heart can be used as an alternative, or a pulse can be felt at the carotid artery which runs alongside the trachea (the windpipe) in the neck.

Factors that can affect the pulse are body temperature, haemorrhagic shock from blood or fluid loss, medications such as digoxin, or severe head injury.

Terminology

dysrhythmia an abnormal heart rhythm

tachycardia an abnormally elevated heart rate (more than 100 beats/minute)

bradycardia an abnormally slow heart rate (less than 60 beats/minute)

When a pulse is palpated it is important to determine the following:

rate – the normal range for adults is 60–100 beats/minute (Potter and Perry 1997)

rhythm – a normal pulse rhythm constitutes a regular succession of beats. You should be able to feel if the heart rate is regular or not

amplitude – the strength of the pulse beat. The pulse can feel weak, faint and 'thready', or strong and 'bounding'.

Intervention: assessment of peripheral pulse

Equipment

- Watch with second hand or digital display.
- Black pen.
- Documentation sheets.

Procedure

- Prepare equipment.
- Wash hands.
- Explain procedure to Mr Ellis.

- Ask Mr Ellis to sit or lie down. Make sure he is as comfortable and relaxed as possible, allowing him to rest for a minimum of five minutes if he has been exercising.
- Place tips of first two or middle three fingers over the groove along the thumb side of Mr Ellis wrist and press gently.
- If the pulse is regular count the number of beats in 30 seconds and multiply the total by 2. If it is irregular, count the pulse rate for one full minute.
- Assess pulse amplitude and rhythm.
- Wash hands.
- Record pulse rate on observation chart and document any abnormalities in amplitude and rhythm.
- Inform Mr Ellis of your findings.
- Report any abnormalities or change in observation to a senior colleague.

TIP! **If a patient's peripheral pulse is irregular it is advisable to compare the reading at the radial artery with the apical pulse to establish whether there is a difference. The most accurate method of achieving this is for two nurses to measure the apical beat and the radial pulse simultaneously. This is known as an 'apex-radial recording'.**

Intervention: assessment of apex-radial pulse

Assessment of the apical pulse involves listening to heart sounds with a stethoscope placed over the apex of the heart. At the same time a second nurse measures the radial pulse.

Equipment

- Stethoscope.
- Watch with second hand or digital display.
- Pens of two different colours (as per Trust policy).
- Documentation sheets.

Procedure

- Prepare equipment: request assistance from a nursing colleague.
- Wash hands.

- Explain procedure to Mr Ellis.
- Ask Mr Ellis to lie down.
- Close curtains around bed.
- Expose sternum and left side of chest.
- Place the diaphragm of the stethoscope over the apex of the heart. This is located at the fifth intercostal space, in line with the left mid-clavicle.
- Listen for the double beat heart sounds. These are referred to as S_1 and S_2 heart sounds.
- When your colleague is ready you should commence counting the apical pulse and she should commence counting the radial pulse. One of you, usually the one counting the apex beat, will need to take the lead when starting the counting and timing the procedure. Count the heart rate for one full minute, counting each double apex beat (S_1 and S_2 sound) as one full beat.
- Help Mr Ellis to get dressed.
- Wash hands.
- Record readings on observation chart, using different colours for the radial and apex measurements, and document any abnormalities in rhythm.
- Inform Mr Ellis of your findings.
- Report any abnormalities or change in observation to a senior colleague.

Blood pressure

Monitoring blood pressure gives an indication of peripheral vascular resistance, the effectiveness of cardiac output, and the amount of blood volume. When measuring the blood pressure two readings are recorded. First, the systolic pressure is measured. This is the pressure that is produced in the arteries when the left ventricle contracts, pushing blood into the aorta. The diastolic pressure is the pressure in the arteries when the heart is in 'diastole' (i.e. relaxes between beats).

Terminology

hypertension blood pressure raised above normal values for the patient's age and condition

hypotension blood pressure lower than normal values

Intervention: taking and recording blood pressure

Record Mr Ellis's blood pressure every *x* minutes. To assess blood pressure using a mercury sphygmomanometer, the British Hypertension Society (Beevers et al. 2001) recommends the following procedure.

Equipment

- Stethoscope.
- Sphygmomanometer with appropriately sized cuff
- Pen and documentation sheets.

Procedure

- Prepare equipment.

ALERT!

The bladder of the cuff should cover 80 per cent of the circumference of the upper arm. Obese or emaciated patients will therefore require large or small cuffs.

- Explain the procedure to Mr Ellis. Ensure that he understands that he should not speak whilst his blood pressure is being measured since this may give a falsely high reading.
- Ask Mr Ellis to sit or lie down. If a comparison between standing and lying blood pressure is required, record the lying blood pressure first.
- Ensure that Mr Ellis is comfortable. To prevent an artificially raised measurement, provide at least 30 minutes, rest after eating or alcohol or caffeine intake.
- When selecting an arm for cuff placement, avoid using an arm affected by an intravenous cannula, an arteriovenous shunt, trauma, full or partial paralysis, or the side of a mastectomy as these conditions will affect the recording and may be painful.
- Wash hands.
- Remove any restrictive clothing from the chosen arm. If it is necessary for Mr Ellis to remove his upper garments provide privacy.

- Position Mr Ellis's arm horizontally, and supported so that the cuff will be level with the heart, palm facing upwards.
- Palpate the brachial artery (this is found in the bend/antecubital fossa of the arm).
- Position the cuff so that the centre of the bladder is over the brachial artery. The lower edge of the cuff should be 2–3 cm above the point of maximum pulsation of the brachial artery. Wrap deflated cuff evenly around upper arm with the rubber tubing from the bladder placed so that it is exiting from the top of the cuff, allowing easy access to the antecubital fossa for auscultation.
- Position manometer at eye level and no further than 3 ft (92 cm) away, so that the scale can be easily read.
- Palpate the brachial artery while inflating the cuff to 30 mmHg above the point where pulsation disappears. Slowly deflate the cuff, noting the pressure at which the pulse reappears. This is the approximate level of the systolic blood pressure. Deflate the cuff. Estimating how high to inflate the cuff by feeling the pulse is important, since phase I sounds (see Table 2.1) may disappear as pressure is reduced and reappear at a lower level.
- Place the diaphragm of the stethoscope over the brachial artery at the point of maximal pulsation. The stethoscope should not touch the cuff, clothing or rubber tubes as this may cause friction sounds. Rapidly inflate the cuff to 30 mmHg above the palpated systolic value. Slowly deflate the cuff at 2–3 mmHg per second. The first Korotkoff sound is the systolic blood pressure. The disappearance of sounds represents the diastolic pressure.
- Record blood pressure on observation chart to the nearest 2 mmHg, noting arm used and position of Mr Ellis. Document any abnormalities or changes.
- Help Mr Ellis to get dressed if necessary and to assume a more comfortable position.
- Wash hands.
- Inform Mr Ellis of your findings.
- Report any abnormalities or change in observation to a senior colleague.

Note If this is the patient's first attendance, his blood pressure should be recorded in both arms (Beevers et al. 2001).

Table 2.1 Korotkoff sounds (adapted from O'Brien and Fitzgerald 1991)

Phase I	The first appearance of faint, clear tapping sounds which gradually increase in intensity for at least two consecutive beats in the systolic blood pressure.
Phase II	A brief period may follow during which the sounds soften and acquire a swishing quality.
Auscultatory gap	In some patients sounds may disappear completely for a short time.
Phase III	The return of sharper sounds, which become crisper to regain or exceed the intensity of phase I sounds.
Phase IV	The distinct, abrupt muffling of sounds, which become soft and blowing.
Phase V	The point at which all sounds disappear.

Avoiding errors in blood pressure measurement

There are various factors that commonly cause errors when measuring a patient's blood pressure. These can be to do with the patient, the nurse, or the equipment.

If a patient is in pain, anxious, or cold, blood pressure will be affected. Try to make sure that the patient does not have a full bladder, and has not had a meal or a cigarette recently. When taking blood pressure, make sure the patient's arm is both horizontal and supported, and that it is not restricted by tight clothing.

As the nurse carrying out this procedure, take care not to round up figures inaccurately, and do not guess at the pressure. Make sure that the cuff and manometer are correctly positioned, and do not deflate the cuff rapidly. Further errors can be caused if a nurse has poor hearing, or fails to interpret Korotkoff sounds accurately.

Check your equipment. The following factors are sources of error: the mercury is not set to zero; the glass is dirty; numbers on the manometer are not clearly visible; equipment may be tilted, or not correctly calibrated or positioned; there may be a defective control valve, or leaks due to cracked or perished rubber tubing.

Aneroid and automated devices

To assess blood pressure using an aneroid sphygmomanometer or an automated device, the cuff should be applied as described above. The aneroid device is used similarly, although the position of the dial is not as important. In using an automated device it is essential that the manufacturer's instructions are followed, as each device will function differently.

Interpretation of results

Clinical management should never be based on a single blood pressure reading (Beevers et al. 2001). The average normal blood pressure for a young adult is 120/80 mmHg; for an older adult it is 140/90 (Potter and Perry 1997).

Body temperature

Core body temperature is controlled by the hypothalamus. Normally, body temperature remains relatively constant, fluctuating only 0.6°C from the average core body temperature of 36°C to 38°C (Perry and Potter 1998). Temperature is affected by:

- infection
- prolonged exposure to heat or cold
- burns
- altered white cell count
- certain drugs
- reactions to blood products
- exercise
- hormonal changes
- damage to the hypothalamus/brain stem.

Body temperature can be assessed at a variety of sites. In intensive care settings, core body temperature can be monitored via the pulmonary artery, oesophagus and bladder. It is more usual for the oral, axillary, rectal or tympanic routes to be used to approximate core body temperature. There are advantages and disadvantages to each of these locations, but to gain an accurate measurement of body temperature it is essential that the chosen route is used correctly.

Terminology

pyrexia   fever, temperature above normal values
hyperpyrexia excessively high temperature above 40°C
hypothermia   temperature below 34.4°C
afebrile   without a fever

Average normal temperature varies according to the measurement site used. The average reading for adults are as follows:

- oral temperature: 37°C
- rectal site: 37.5°C
- axilla site: 36.5°C
- tympanic route: 36.8–37.9°C (Braun et al. 1998; Perry and Potter 1998).

Throughout the UK, the majority of Trusts are phasing out mercury thermometers and replacing them with electronic devices. This reflects concerns over potential mercury spillages, reduction in cross-infection from using disposable probe covers, and more rapid readings from electronic devices than mercury thermometers.

Electronic thermometers

The position for recording a patient's temperature using an electronic thermometer is the same as a mercury thermometer for each of the sites. However, the manufacturer's guidelines should always be followed concerning the amount of time that the probe is left in situ and preparing, activating and cleaning the device.

Intervention: taking and recording body temperature

Record Mr Ellis's temperature every *x* minutes.

Measuring oral temperature

Note The oral site would be inappropriate for Mr Ellis due to his altered level of consciousness.

Advantages of oral route

- Easily accessible.
- Placement of the thermometer directly above the sublingual artery, which is proximal to the external carotid artery, allows changes in core temperature to be reflected promptly (Watson 1998).

Disadvantages

- Accuracy of the reading may be affected by ingestion of fluids or foods, smoking, oxygen delivery and mouth breathing (Braun et al. 1998).
- This site is not suitable if the patient is unable to hold the thermometer in position or when the thermometer may cause injury – for example, in patients who have mouth pain or trauma; confused or unconscious patients; people with a history of convulsions; and patients with rigors. It is also contraindicated for people who need to breathe through their mouths, since airflow will affect the accuracy of the result (Braun et al. 1998).
- Risk of body fluid exposure.

Equipment

- Mercury thermometer/electronic thermometer.
- Disposable cover (depending upon hospital policy).
- Pen and documentation sheets.
- Disinfection materials for cleaning the thermometer in accordance with local policy.

Procedure

- Assess whether it is safe to use the oral site.
- Ensure that the patient has not consumed any hot or cold liquids or food, or smoked during the preceding 20 minutes, as this will affect the accuracy of the measurement (Braun et al. 1998).
- Prepare equipment.
- Explain the procedure to the patient, ensuring that he understands the importance of maintaining correct position of the thermometer.
- Wash hands.

Glass thermometer:

- Holding the glass end of the thermometer in your fingertips, read the mercury level.
- If the mercury level is greater than 35.5°C shake the mercury down by flicking the wrist downwards until it is below 35°C.
- Apply disposable cover.
- Ask the patient to open his mouth, and place the silver bulb of the thermometer in the sublingual pocket, on either side of the frenulum below the tongue.
- Ask the patient to hold the thermometer with lips closed; this will ensure that the thermometer remains in the correct position.
- Leave the thermometer in place for a minimum of 2 minutes (Torrance and Semple 1998).
- Remove the thermometer, remove cover and read at eye level.
- Inform patient of reading and document measurement.
- Report any changes to senior colleague.
- Clean thermometer according to local policy.

TIP! **Each patient should be allocated his own glass thermometer or probe cover to prevent cross-infection.**
If mercury thermometers are used in your clinical area ensure that you know how to clear up a mercury spill should a mercury thermometer break.

Measuring rectal temperature

Advantages

- It used to be argued that the main advantage of this site was that it was safe for use in the unconscious patient and it was relatively accurate. Although the rectal route reflects core body temperature more accurately than the axillary site it is now rarely used, since tympanic measurement has been found to be less expensive (Stavem et al. 2000) and just as accurate (Cronin and Wallis 2000).

Disadvantages

- Potentially embarrassing and uncomfortable for patients.
- Unsuitable for patients who have had rectal surgery or a rectal disorder.

- Risk of body fluid exposure.
- Inferior to the oral and tympanic site in reflecting changes in core temperature, since it is a cavity and can therefore retain heat longer than other sites (Severine and McKenzie 1997).

Equipment

- Glass rectal tip mercury thermometer (rectal thermometers are marked with a blue tip) or electronic thermometer with rectal probe.
- Disposable cover.
- Water-soluble lubricant.
- Tissues.
- Pen and documentation sheets.
- Disinfection materials for cleaning the thermometer in accordance with local Trust policy.

Procedure

- Assess whether it is appropriate to use the rectal site (see advantages and disadvantages above).
- Prepare equipment.
- Explain the procedure to the patient.
- Draw curtains around bed.
- Position patient on his side, in the left lateral position if possible, with upper legs flexed. Keep body fully covered, ensuring that anal area can be easily exposed.
- Wash hands and apply disposable gloves.

Glass thermometer:

- Holding the glass end of the thermometer in your fingertips, read the mercury level.
- If the mercury level is greater than 35.5°C shake the mercury down by flicking the wrist downward until it is below 35°C.
- Apply disposable cover.
- Apply lubricant onto a tissue. Dip tapered end of thermometer into lubricant, covering up to 5 cm; this minimizes trauma to the rectal mucosa.
- Expose rectal area. With non-dominant hand raise client's upper buttock to expose anus.

- Ask patient to take deep breaths, to relax the anal sphincter. As the patient exhales, gently insert thermometer 5 cm into anus, towards the umbilicus (Severine and McKenzie 1997). If there is any resistance, withdraw the thermometer.
- Hold the thermometer in place for a minimum of 3 minutes (Torrance and Semple 1998).
- Remove the thermometer, remove cover and read at eye level.
- Wipe client's anal area to remove lubricant and/or faeces.
- Remove gloves and wash hands.
- Help patient to replace clothing and to resume a more comfortable position.
- Inform patient of reading, and document measurement, clearly indicating that the rectal site has been used.
- Report any changes to senior colleague.
- Clean thermometer according to local policy.

TIP! Always hold the thermometer in place – sudden movement could cause the thermometer to break.

If hypothermia is suspected, a low-reading thermometer should be used.

Measuring axillary temperature

Advantages

- Non-invasive.

Disadvantages

- Takes a longer time to achieve an accurate reading.
- Less accurate than other sites, because: the axilla is not close to any major vessels; skin temperature varies with changes in the environment, and readings will be affected by peripheral vasoconstriction.

Equipment

- Glass mercury thermometer/electronic thermometer.
- Pen and documentation sheets.
- Disinfection materials for cleaning the thermometer in accordance with local trust policy.

Procedure

- Assess whether an alternative site could be used (see advantages and disadvantages above).
- Prepare equipment.
- Explain the procedure to the patient.
- Draw curtains around bed.
- Position patient in a sitting or supine position. Keep body fully covered, ensuring axillary area can be easily accessed.
- Ensure axilla is dry.
- Wash hands.

Glass thermometer:

- Holding the glass end of the thermometer in your fingertips, read the mercury level.
- If the mercury level is greater than 35.5°C, shake the mercury down by flicking the wrist downwards until it is below 35°C.
- Place thermometer into centre of patient's axilla; ask patient to lower his arm over the thermometer and place forearm across his chest, in order to keep thermometer in correct position.
- Hold the thermometer in place for a minimum of 5 minutes (Torrance and Semple 1998).
- Remove the thermometer and read at eye level.
- Help patient to replace clothing and to resume a more comfortable position.
- Wash hands.
- Inform patient of reading, and document measurement, clearly indicating that the axillary site has been used.
- Report any changes to senior colleague.
- Clean thermometer according to local policy.

Measuring tympanic temperature

Advantages

- Readily accessible.
- Provides accurate core reading because of the tympanic membrane's proximity to the hypothalamus and its shared blood supply with the hypothalamus via the internal carotid arteries (Severine and McKenzie 1997).

- Rapid measurement.
- Limited exposure to body fluids.

Disadvantages

- Requires removal of hearing aids.
- Unsuitable for patients who have had ear surgery, or who have blood or fluid present within ear canal.
- Readings may be distorted if there is earwax (cerumen), or if otitis media is present.

Equipment

- Tympanic thermometer with disposable ear cover.
- Pen and documentation sheets.

Procedure

- Assess whether this site is suitable.
- Prepare equipment.
- Explain the procedure to the patient.
- Place disposable cover on the thermometer.
- Expose patient's external auditory canal, and insert probe by pulling the pinna up and back; this straightens the external auditory canal, exposing the tympanic membrane. Fit probe snugly into the canal so that it is occluded. This will eliminate the effect of airflow into the canal, which can have a significant effect on the accuracy of the reading (Braun et al. 1998).
- Hold the thermometer in place until a reading is displayed on the digital unit.
- Dispose of probe cover.
- Wash hands.
- Inform patient of reading, and document measurement, clearly indicating that the tympanic site has been used.
- Report any changes to senior colleague.

Assessing level of consciousness

The Glasgow Coma Scale (Figure 2.1), used in conjunction with vital signs, is frequently used to assess a patient's level of consciousness. The scale uses three indicators of consciousness: eye opening, motor response and verbal response. A score is awarded for the patient's performance in each area.

Observations

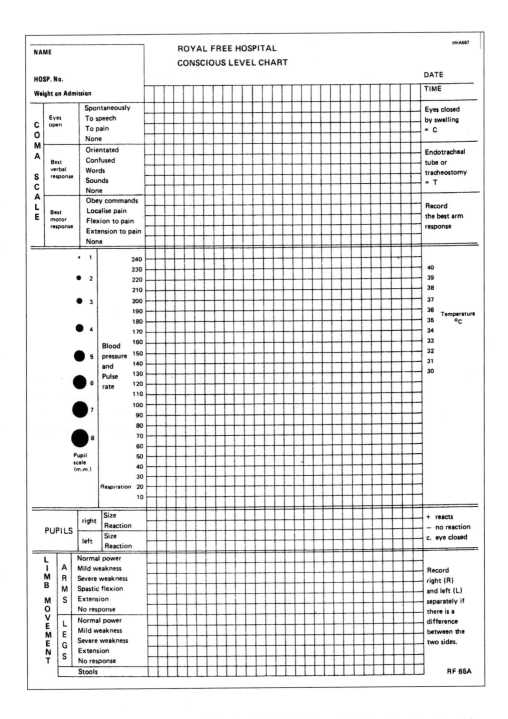

Figure 2.1 Conscious level chart (copied with kind permission from Royal Free Hospital NHS Trust).

The level of consciousness may be assessed by a variety of methods. Explain to the patient, whether they are conscious or unconscious, that frequent observations are needed, both during the day and night. It is widely believed that unconscious patients continue to hear sounds even if they cannot respond, and if explanations are not given, they may become restless and distressed.

All observations should be recorded according to local documentation.

Intervention: assessment of level of consciousness

Assess Mr Ellis's level of consciousness every x minutes.

Equipment

- A pen torch.
- Glasgow Coma Scale Chart.
- Equipment for vital sign assessment, as detailed above.

TIP! **Before assessing a patient's level of consciousness, it is important to assess him for sedation by medication or other substances, paralysis, spinal cord injury, language barriers or degrees of deafness as these will affect his ability to respond.**

Procedure to assess eye-opening response

This response is assessed according to the following criteria:

'*Opens eyes spontaneously*': eyes will open without any stimulation from the observer such as speech or touch. This can be seen from a distance. If the patient is unable to open an eye because of oedema, nerve palsy or the presence of an eye dressing this should be documented. If the eyes are open and no blinking is apparent, gently close the eyes and see if they open spontaneously.

'*Eyes open to verbal stimuli*': if eye opening does not occur spontaneously, talk to the patient and note the response. Initially, approach the patient and greet him by name, without touching him. If there is no response, proceed to ask the patient to open his eyes. If there is still no response, raise your voice and repeat the instruction.

'*Eyes open to pain*': if there is no response to speech, touch the patient's hand or shoulder or gently shake him. If this does not elicit a response, apply light pressure to the trapezius (muscle at the base of the neck to the top of the shoulder), gently rub the sternum, or apply light pressure to the supraorbital region. This technique and others are discussed in more detail below (page 38; see also Lowry 1998).

ALERT!

See guidelines in 'pain response' about testing a patient's response to pain. This procedure should be used with caution to prevent injury.

'*None*': the patient fails to open his eyes. This may indicate injury to the oculomotor nerve or the brain stem.

Procedure to assess verbal response

This response is assessed according to the following criteria:

'*Makes orientated speech*': if the patient is able to accurately describe details of time, person and place he is said to be orientated (Jennett and Teasdale 1974; Aucken and Crawford 1998).

'*Makes confused speech*': at this level the patient is able to form sentences (he may also have a good attention span and be able to engage in conversation), but is unable to answer questions that show he is orientated in time, place or person (Aucken and Crawford 1998).

'*Inappropriate words*': this category may be appropriate when the patient cannot converse; when there is a tendency to use words rather then sentences; when replies are only forthcoming following painful stimulation; when words or phrases are repeated; or when there is consistent loss of attention.

TIP! A patient whose first language is not English may revert to his mother tongue so appearing confused. An interpreter may be of assistance.

'Incomprehensible sounds': the patient responds to stimuli or spontaneously makes sounds rather than uses words.

'None': no sounds at all are made regardless of stimuli. If this is due to
the presence of an endotracheal or tracheostomy tube this should
be noted.

Procedure to assess motor response

This response is assessed according to the following criteria:

ALERT!

**Using a painful stimulus is highly contentious when
determining a patient's neurological status and should
only be used with *great caution* (Lowry 1998).**

'Obeys commands': the patient is able to obey simple commands, such
as 'Lift up your right arm'.

'Localizes to pain': if the patient is unable to obey simple commands, a
central pain stimulus should be applied briefly. 'Localizing to pain'
is said to occur when a patient raises his hand to at least chin
level, when the painful stimulus is above that level, e.g. trapezius
pinch or supraorbital ridge pressure, or when he tries to remove
the painful stimulus.

Suggested techniques for applying central painful stimuli are:

- supraorbital ridge pressure: place hand on patient's forehead,
  applying the flat of your thumb on the supraorbital ridge (the
  bony ridge along the top of the eye). Gradually increase the pressure until there is a response or maximum pressure exerted. Do *not*
  apply prolonged pressure or use repeatedly as this can result in
  tissue damage. This site should *not* be used if orbital damage or
  facial or skull fractures are present (Lowry 1998; Shah 1999).
- trapezius pinch: expose the shoulder and pinch the trapezius
  muscle gently. This muscle is located at the base of the neck,
  running to the shoulder. Gradually increase the pressure until a
  response is elicited or maximum pressure exerted. Do *not* apply

prolonged pressure or use repeatedly as this can result in tissue damage (Lowry 1998; Shah 1999).

Note **Rubbing the sternum or applying pressure to the fingers or nailbeds is not recommended since this may cause lasting tissue damage (Lowry 1998).**

'Normal flexion to pain': arms bend upwards at the elbows, without wrist rotation, as a response to pain (Figure 2.2.1) (Shah 1999).

'Abnormal flexion to pain': arms bend outwards from elbows, with wrist rotated resulting in spastic posture, as a response to pain (Figure 2.2.2) (Shah 1999).

'Extends to pain': arms extend at the elbows, rotating inwards, following pain stimulus (Figure 2.2.3) (Shah 1999).

'No response': no response is observed following the application of painful stimuli.

Procedure to assess pupil reaction and size

If intra-cranial pressure is rising within the skull, the optic nerve may be compressed, interfering with the pupil's normal reaction to light.

To assess the size of the patient's pupils, observe the size of each pupil. Relate to the diagrams provided on the observation chart and record the appropriate size for each eye. This observation should be performed before direct light is applied to the eyes (see below).

To assess pupil reaction, dim the light in the room, hold the patient's eyelid open and slowly move the light from the torch across the patient's pupil and beyond, watching closely for a change in pupil size (Lowry 1998). Repeat on other eye. Record whether each pupil constricted briskly, sluggishly or failed to react on the observation chart as per the local documentation.

Procedure to assess motor function/limb movement in upper limbs

For the conscious patient, hold the patient's hands one at a time and ask him to push you away or pull you towards him, while you apply some resistance. Assess the power and equality of movement to determine whether either side is weaker than the other. Document your observations using the categories in Table 2.2, p. 41.

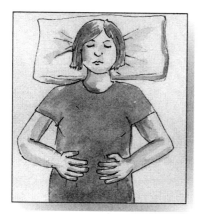

Figure 2.2.1.
Normal flexion.

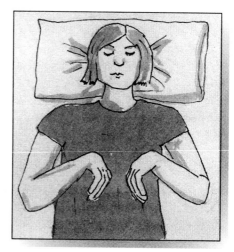

Figure 2.2.2
Abnormal flexion.

Figure 2.2.3
Abnormal extension.

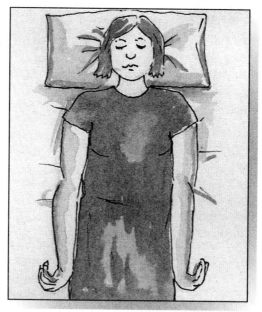

Figure 2.2.1–3 Assessing motor response.

For the unconscious patient the earlier responses to painful stimuli should be documented (see Table 2.2).

Procedure to assess motor function/limb movement in lower limbs

For the conscious patient, place resistance on the patient's knees and ask him to lift his knees up. Assess the power and equality of movement. Record your observations using the categories detailed in Table 2.2.

For the unconscious patient the earlier responses to pain should be recorded (see Table 2.2). Record your observations using the categories below. You will note that on the observation chart (Figure 2.1) spastic flexion is not included in the list for legs; this is because flexion of the legs to pain is a normal response. Spontaneous movement in any limb in an unconscious patient should be noted, even if it is not in response to external stimuli.

Table 2.2 Categories for assessment of motor function (Shah 1999)

Normal power	Able to match resistance applied allowing for age and build
Mild weakness	Able to move limb against resistance but is easily overcome
Severe weakness	Unable to move limb against resistance
Spastic flexion	Flexion at the elbow
Extension	Extension of the limb in response to pain
No response	Patient responds to none of the above

Vital signs

It is important that the patient's temperature, heart rate, blood pressure and respiratory rate are also recorded since alterations in vital signs may indicate compression or damage within the brain stem.

TIP! **At nursing handover it is good practice for a set of neurological observations to be carried out by the handover nurse with the next nurse present to ensure consistency of results.**

Blood glucose levels

Disorders of blood glucose levels affect the ability of the brain to function normally. Causes vary but include:

- poorly controlled diabetes mellitus
- starvation
- physiological stress
- renal, hepatic or pancreatic disease
- endocrine disturbances.

Any patient who presents with an altered level of consciousness should have his blood glucose levels checked to exclude hypoglycaemia.

Intervention: measuring blood glucose levels

Measure Mr Ellis's blood glucose levels every x hours.

Equipment

- Glucose meter (if available).
- Disposable finger pricking device or lancet.
- Gauze swab/cotton-wool ball.
- Disposable injection tray.
- Blood glucose testing strips.
- Disposable gloves.
- Pen and documentation sheets.

Procedure

- Prepare equipment.
- Explain procedure to Mr Ellis.
- Ask Mr Ellis to wash his hands or assist him to do so.

TIP! **Do not use alcohol swabs to clean the patient's finger as this alters the result and causes cracking of the patient's skin.**

- Wash your hands and apply protective gloves.
- Select an appropriate finger for the procedure. Sites should be rotated. It is important that an insulin or glucose infusion is not

in progress on the side chosen for obtaining the reading since this may give a misleading result.

- Check expiry date of testing strips and prepare glucose measurement meter according to the manufacturer's instructions.
- Ask Mr Ellis to hold his hand down to encourage circulation to the fingers. Using the appropriate device, prick the side of his fingertip.
- Place the used lancet onto the injection tray for disposal.
- Direct the drop of blood onto the testing strip, taking care to let the blood drop onto the strip rather than smearing it on.
- Follow the manufacturer's instructions with regard to how long to leave the blood on the strip, and to use of the meter.
- Assist Mr Ellis to gently apply pressure to the site, using the cotton wool or gauze to stop bleeding and prevent bruising.
- Read the result from the meter when the meter indicates that the result is available, or, if using a manual technique, match the colour of the strip to that given on the container after the appropriate time.
- Dispose of sharps; remove gloves and wash hands.
- Document observation, inform Mr Ellis of the implications of the reading, and inform a senior colleague of the result.

ALERT!

If using a meter, it is vital to check it for accuracy before use. Incorrect readings can cause incorrect management, which could be fatal. It is recommended that quality control checks are made daily and when starting a fresh batch of test strips.

Measure Mr Ellis's respiratory rate and oxygen saturation levels

Please refer to Chapter 8.

An additional method of assessment that is beyond the scope of this introductory text is ECG monitoring. This requires additional training and advanced skills.

Evaluation

Were Mr Ellis's observations monitored and recorded accurately? Were any abnormalities detected and reported?

Further reading

Lowry M (1998) Trauma, emergency nursing and the Glasgow Coma Scale. Accident and Emergency Nursing 6(3): 143–48.

Watson R (1998) Controlling body temperature in adults. Nursing Standard 12(20): 49–55.

Principles of caring

CHAPTER 3

Infection control

Barbara Workman

Aims and learning outcomes

This chapter introduces the essential principles of preventing the transmission of infection. By the end of this chapter you will be able to:

- outline universal infection control precautions
- describe three types of handwashing procedure and state when to use each one
- explain what to do if a needlestick injury occurs
- identify procedures that require the use of protective clothing
- describe how to dispose of waste safely.

Preventing transmission of infection

Patients are at risk of infection from their own resident micro-organisms (endogenous infection), or from external micro-organisms (exogenous infection), which may result from transmission from infected patients, carriers or equipment during their treatment. Health care workers' hands are also known to be the main source of transmission, and efforts to prevent transmission of infection between patients and staff during the course of treatment should be made (Department of Health 2001a).

A recent government report (Mayor 2000) indicated that as many as 5 000 patients die as a result of hospital-acquired infections

(HAI) every year. The full impact of HAI cannot be fully calculated since this type of infection has hidden costs, such as the following:

- prolonged hospitalization
- increased pain and discomfort
- additional loss of earnings
- increased intake of medications with potential side effects
- extended disruption to the patient's lifestyle and family
- lengthened recovery time.

Identifiable costs to the health care trust include the use of more equipment such as protective clothing, additional treatment time and length of admission, and the use of more expert services such as microbiology and infection control staff (Ayliffe et al. 1999).

Nurses must ensure that good infection control practices are maintained, always 'acting in a manner to promote and safe guard the interests and well-being of patients' (UKCC 1992), thereby protecting their patients from acquiring infections from any potential source. A common problem in hospitals is the spread of Methicillin-resistant *Staphylococcus aureus* (MRSA), a bacterium resistant to the majority of known antibiotics, which therefore causes virulent infections in susceptible patients. This is a worldwide problem, and is made more difficult to control as the bacteria develop different strains over time, and emerge differently in various locations (Ayliffe et al. 1999). The principles of preventing infection are therefore as important as dealing with a known infection, as prevention is always better than cure.

To be able to prevent infection spreading from one person to another the 'chain of infection' (May 2001) has to be broken (Figure 3.1). Taking appropriate precautions at any stage of the chain will reduce the risks of infection spreading.

Source/reservoir → Route of → Susceptible → Point of
of micro-   transmission   host   entry
organism

Figure 3.1 Chain of infection.

NURSING PROBLEM 3.1

Problem: Health care staff at risk of infection from blood-borne viruses and direct and indirect patient contacts.

Goal: Staff will not acquire infection.

Principles of universal infection control precautions

Universal infection control precautions (UICP) are practices that are applied to all patients to reduce transmission of a blood-borne disease – such as Human Immunodeficiency Virus (HIV) or Hepatitis B or C – to either a health care worker or another patient. As it is impossible to know which patients may be infected without taking a blood test, it is recommended that all patients should be considered potential hazards (RCN 1997). The most likely means of transmission is by a sharps injury, or by blood or body fluid splashing directly onto a mucous membrane or into eyes, and therefore routine measures should be taken to protect staff and patients. Application of UICP to all patient care will also reduce the spread of MRSA before it is confirmed by laboratory results.

The aims of universal infection control precautions are to:

- prevent blood or body fluids from coming into contact with broken skin, or mucous membranes
- minimize blood or body fluid contact with intact skin
- prevent sharps injuries
- protect staff against Hepatitis B and C
- prevent contaminated items being used between patients (Ayliffe et al. 1999).

Routine precautions

There are various routine precautions that should always be taken:

- It is your personal responsibility to ensure your Hepatitis B vaccination is kept up to date.

- Handwashing is essential before, between and after patient contact (Figure 3.2).
- Skin: broken skin should be covered by a waterproof dressing that acts as a barrier to micro-organisms; avoid invasive procedures if you have chronic skin wounds.
- Gloves should be worn during procedures that carry risk of contamination by blood or body fluids (see below).
- Protective clothing such as aprons should be worn to reduce contamination (see below).
- Mucous membranes of eyes, mouth and nose should be protected from blood or body fluid splashes, e.g. protective spectacles may be used during tracheal suction. If contamination occurs irrigate with saline solution and follow steps 4–6 below.
- Know the procedure for dealing with a needlestick injury. Concentrate and do not rush during procedures, to prevent this occurring.

TIP! **It is rare for a needlestick injury to occur, or for it to result in a serious infection, but make sure you know the steps to take if it happens. Do not be tempted to leave it to deal with later because you are busy. It is the Trust's responsibility to provide a specialist practitioner within your Trust, who will be able to assess your risk of becoming infected and provide appropriate advice and support (UK Health Departments 1998).**

Disposal of sharps

Sharps should be used and disposed of with extreme care:

- take personal responsibility for disposing of sharps you have used immediately after use
- never resheath needles
- dispose of sharps as near to place of use as possible
- do not overfill sharps containers (they should be no more than two-thirds full).

Actions in case of a sharps injury

1. Encourage wound to bleed, do not suck.

2. Wash the area with warm water, and soap or antiseptic agent thoroughly.
3. Cover with waterproof dressing.
4. If known note the name of the patient.
5. Report immediately to occupational health department if during office hours, or designated location (e.g. Accident and Emergency) out of hours. This will enable you to take post-exposure prophylaxis for HIV and Hepatitis B.
6. Notify your line manager and document the incident (UK Health Department 1998).

Spillages of blood or body fluids

Blood spillages require treatment either with hypochlorite solution (e.g. Domestos or Milton) or Sodium dichloroisocyanurates (NaDCC), which are chlorine-releasing agents (e.g. Precept or Haz tabs), before the area is cleaned as directed by local Infection Control protocols (UK Health Department 1998).

Intervention

- Clear up spillages of body fluids immediately.
- Wearing gloves and apron, either wipe up spillage with paper towels or, if the surface is suitable, cover with NaDCC granules.
- Allow a few minutes to elapse.
- Clear towels or granules and dispose in clinical waste bag (usually yellow).
- Clean with hypochlorite solution.

Waste

Use correct colour coding for domestic and clinical waste. The usual colour coding in the UK is:

- black or clear bags for domestic and household waste
- yellow bags for clinical waste, including human or animal tissue, excreta, blood or body fluids, or pharmaceutical products
- glass, aerosols and sharps are disposed of separately.

Waste bags and containers are to be labelled indicating the clinical area they originated from to enable tracing if necessary.

Laundry

This should also be bagged in colour-coded bags:

● white bags for used and soiled linen
● red outer bag for blood-stained and infectious linen, to warn laundry staff that it is potentially hazardous.

TIP! **When cleaning up after a procedure or emergency make sure sharps are not inadvertently discarded in bed linen – this causes additional hazards for laundry staff.**

NURSING PROBLEM 3.2

Patient history: Mrs Gray is an elderly lady admitted to the ward with a fractured femur that has been fixed with a pin and plate.

Problem: Mrs Gray is at risk of developing a hospital-acquired infection (HAI).

Goal: Mrs Gray will not develop an HAI.

Preventing infection transmission between staff and/or patients

Handwashing

Effective handwashing is absolutely essential in preventing cross-infection, and aims to remove dirt and micro-organisms from the hands. Studies (Department of Health 2001a) showed that effective handwashing significantly reduces the transmission of HAI. The use of suitable antiseptic lotions and brisk rubbing will remove temporary and resident organisms and leave the hands disinfected.

Handwashing schedule

The following schedule indicates some key times when handwashing is obligatory.

Before:

- direct patient contact or care of immuno-compromised patients
- handling food, pouring drinks or dispensing medicine
- aseptic procedures such as wound care
- invasive procedures such as caring for an intravenous site
- touching wounds or dressings
- entering isolation rooms
- leaving the clinical area for another location.

After:

- leaving isolation rooms
- touching wounds or dressings
- contact with or disposal of blood or body fluids, secretions or ex-creta: e.g. bedpans, urinals, suction equipment
- removing gloves
- touching equipment contaminated by body fluids, e.g. urine test-ing equipment, sputum pots
- caring for patients known to be colonized with bacteria, e.g. Methicillin-resistant *Staphylococcus aureus* (MRSA)
- cleaning and changing beds or surrounding areas
- personal toileting, blowing/touching your nose, or touching your hair (Infection Control Nurses Association 1997).

TIP! A good guide as to when hands need washing is to imagine that you are about to eat a meal with your fingers! If your hands are not clean enough to eat with, they are not clean enough to care for a patient or touch his environment.

Ayliffe et al. (1999) describe three types of handwashing procedure: social handwash, hygienic hand disinfection, and surgical scrub.

Social handwash

This is the most common form of handwash and should be used

following activities such as direct patient contact, blowing the nose, toileting, and prior to preparing food.

To clean dirt and remove transient organisms from hands, 3–5 ml of liquid soap is used, and washing follows the procedure described below (Intervention: handwashing procedures) for 10–15 seconds. Liquid soap is used instead of bar soap which has been proved to harbour micro-organisms. Drying must be thorough and may be with paper towels or, in the community, a towel designated in the home for the health care worker.

Hand disinfection

Instead of soap, 3–5 ml of antiseptic washing solution such as chlorhexidine, triclosan or providone iodine should be used, for a duration of 15–30 seconds, followed by thorough drying. This removes the vast majority of transient organisms and should be used in all cases where vulnerable patients are cared for, such as immuno-compromised patients, those with MRSA, neonates and those in intensive care. This method should also be used before aseptic procedures such as urinary catheterization or wound dressing.

Surgical scrub

This may be used prior to surgery or invasive procedures: it requires handwashing with 3–5 ml of antiseptic solution for up to two minutes, and includes cleaning the fingernails. The use of an antiseptic agent for this length of time will retain the antibacterial action for longer afterwards. Drying should be with a sterile towel.

TIP! **Communal scrubbing brushes have been found to be a potential source of infection and therefore should not be used.**

Intervention: handwashing procedures

Remove all jewellery, such as rings and bracelets, as it can harbour micro-organisms. It is acceptable to leave a wedding ring on, but advisable to wash and dry beneath it.

1. Using a sink with elbow or foot operated taps is preferable. Adjust the flow until a comfortably warm temperature is achieved and the water is not splashing out of the sink. Wet hands.

2. Apply 3–5 ml of liquid soap or antiseptic solution and follow the six-step pattern (see Figures 3.2.1–6), rubbing briskly.
   1. Rub palm to palm.
   2. Alternate palms over the back of hands.
   3. Interlace fingers palms together, washing between the base of fingers.
   4. Clasp fingers in opposing palms, washing the tops of the fingers.
   5. Alternate thumbs rubbed within opposite palm.
   6. Rub centre of palms with opposite fingertips.

For effective hand disinfection, rub at least five times at each step (Infection Control Nurses Association 1997). For surgical scrub, washing should take at least two minutes and include the forearms and wrists, working downwards from hands towards elbows.

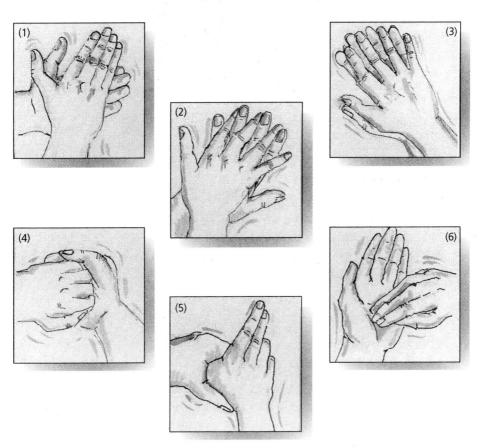

Figure 3.2.1–6 Handwashing.

3. Rinse the hands thoroughly until all traces of detergent are removed, allowing the water to run down the hands, from the fingers pointing upwards (Figure 3.3).

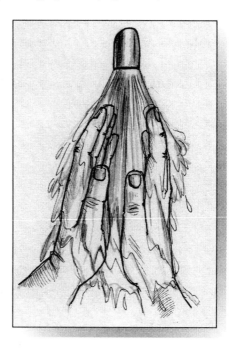

Figure 3.3 Rinsing hands.

4. Turn off the taps with elbow or foot, or use a paper towel to turn off the tap.
5. Dry thoroughly using disposable paper towels, working from fingers downwards, one hand at a time. Ensure all areas are dry to prevent chapping.
6. Dispose of towels in waste bin as directed by local policy, e.g. either as household rubbish (black bag) or clinical waste (yellow).

Alcohol hand rubs

Physically clean hands can be disinfected with 5 ml of alcohol rub, using the six-step technique for routine handwashing if quick disinfection is required or there are poor washing facilities. Alcohol is ineffective if dirt is present. Two applications of alcohol rub are required prior to surgical procedures (Ayliffe et al. 1999).

TIP! Frequent handwashing may result in dry and sore hands. Make sure that hands are dried thoroughly and do not use antiseptic solutions for routine social washing. If you use a hand lotion, use a personal dispenser or hand pump device, which can be discarded when empty. This reduces bacterial growth and prevents contamination between individuals.

Gloves

If gloves are to protect the wearer then non-sterile gloves will usually be appropriate, as they protect from heavy contamination during procedures, and prevent staff–patient and patient–patient cross-infection. Gloves are *not* a substitute for handwashing: they provide a warm, moist environment that encourages bacteria to grow, and may be penetrated by external bacteria. Furthermore, indiscriminate wearing of gloves may cause adverse reactions and skin sensitivity. Be sure, therefore, to wear gloves at the right time and for the right reasons. For example: gloves are not necessary when helping a patient onto a bedpan; to protect yourself from body fluids, however, wear gloves when removing a bedpan. Sterile gloves are necessary for invasive procedures and most procedures involving immuno-compromised patients. Check your local policies when choosing and using gloves.

TIP! To reduce the likelihood of developing allergy to gloves, use powder-free gloves, and wash and dry hands thoroughly after use.

Gloves should be worn:

- only once, and should not be washed for reuse
- when in contact with blood, body fluids or excreta
- when handling soiled or contaminated equipment or linen
- when caring for patients with a known infection, such as MRSA.

Gloves should be discarded:

- between each patient
- if they become heavily soiled, or contaminated with infected material
- if torn during patient care.

Aprons

Protective clothing is worn to reduce transmission of micro-organisms between patients or when there is a risk that clothing or uniform may become exposed to blood, body fluids, secretions and excretions, with the exception of sweat (Department of Health 2001a). Plastic aprons protect uniforms more effectively than cotton gowns. Aprons should not be used as a substitute for a daily clean uniform, and ideally uniforms should be laundered by the Trust to ensure adequate cleaning. Home laundering may be insufficient if the uniform has been contaminated with body fluids (Ayliffe et al. 1999).

Situations that require aprons

A clean apron should be worn and then discarded afterwards when:

● bedmaking: ideally, patients known to be infected should have their beds changed last to reduce potential transmission of infection to vulnerable and uninfected patients; if linen is clearly contaminated with body fluids change the apron after handling
● giving total patient care
● assisting toileting
● dispensing food and feeding patients – a special colour-coded apron may be worn for food handling
● cleaning or performing other tasks likely to cause splashing and soiling of uniforms
● involved with aseptic or invasive procedures.

Procedure

● Wash and dry hands.
● Select appropriate colour apron.
● Put apron over head, avoiding contact with hair and uniform.
● Loosely secure apron at the back – this prevents splashes from trickling onto clothing.
● After procedure, break neck and waist ties (Figures 3.4.1–2) by gently pulling apart.
● Fold inwards so that the potentially contaminated front does not touch hands or uniform (Figure 3.4.3).
● Discard into clinical waste bag.
● Wash and dry hands.

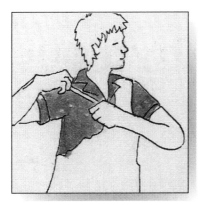

Figure 3.4.1
Break neck tie.

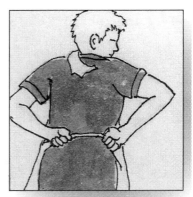

Figure 3.4.2
Break waist tie.

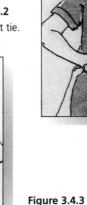

Figure 3.4.3
Fold inwards to
discard.

Figure 3.4.1–3 Removing apron.

Evaluation

Mrs Gray does not acquire an HAI.

Further reading

Ayliffe GAJ, Babb JR, Taylor LJ (1999) Hospital-Acquired Infection: Principles and Prevention, 3rd edn. Oxford: Butterworth-Heinemann.

Department of Health (2001a) Standard principles for preventing hospital-acquired infections. Journal of Hospital Infection 47: S21–S37. See also http://www. idealibrary.com.

CHAPTER 4

Personal hygiene

Frances Gordon

Aims and learning outcomes

This chapter considers how the needs of patients who are unable to undertake their normal hygiene and grooming activities can be met. By the end of this chapter you will be able to:

● understand the importance of hygiene and grooming to a sense of self and personal dignity
● understand how hygiene and grooming contributes to the total health of the patient
● assist a patient to maintain normal grooming habits while confined to bed
● ensure the maintenance of a healthy mouth through adequate mouth care
● promote a return to patient independence in meeting hygiene needs as recovery proceeds.

Personal hygiene needs

Attending to personal hygiene needs can, at first sight, seem a very simple set of activities. Many people care for their children and at times adult members of their family in this way without any special training or preparation. However, ensuring that patients feel clean and comfortable is one of the most important and skilled elements of nursing work. Meeting the hygiene needs of a person who is seriously ill or has restricted mobility can be very challenging. The skills required are vital to a patient's wellbeing and dignity. We all carry notions of what we would ideally wish to look like, and we manage our appearance in ways that take us as near to this ideal as possible. Most adults expect to be able to maintain their own personal hygiene and grooming and to present themselves to the world in ways that satisfy their personal image, and if this ability is compromised, so may be that person's sense of self and dignity. Most of us would feel somewhat alarmed if we had to present ourselves to the public gaze straight from bed without a wash, without cleaning our teeth, without having a shave or putting on make-up, without washing our hair or arranging it as we like, or without being dressed in clothes that we feel suit us. A high standard of hygiene and grooming helps to maintain dignity and a sense of self in vulnerable patients, and reassures their friends and relatives that their loved one is cared for.

Apart from personal presentation, meeting the hygiene needs of ill and dependent patients is vital to the functioning of the body. The skin provides an effective barrier against pathogens and physical forces. Neglected hygiene can increase the incidence of infection and breakdown of the skin and the mucosa of the mouth. This is even more problematic where patients are ill and debilitated and so have depleted body defences against infection. Personal hygiene is a prime marker of the standard of care a patient receives. It provides a line of defence against infection and is therefore important to the patient's physical safety.

How should the professional carer think about planning care that meets the hygiene needs of individual patients? We are all different and all meet our personal hygiene needs according to our acquired behaviours and lifestyle. This can be a sensitive issue when the nurse's and patient's notions of an acceptable standard differ, and will need to be negotiated by listening to and respecting the patient's views. Making an assessment of the patient's normal grooming habits and considering the additional needs imposed by his illness are an appropriate starting point. For instance, a patient who is perspiring freely because of his illness may require additional access to washing facilities compared to his normal daily washing activities. People who take a daily shower but have mobility problems that confine them to bed will need to have a daily all-over wash by methods that can be used at the bedside.

The following classes of patients are likely to need assistance with their hygiene and grooming needs:

- people with limited mobility or restricted movement
- patients with pain that is debilitating
- unconscious patients
- patients with cognitive problems, such as confused older people.

Patient history

Mrs Jenny Brown has been admitted to a general medical ward via the Accident and Emergency Department. Mrs Brown is 74 years old and has had a stroke that has left her with a one-sided paralysis. Mrs Brown is conscious but at present is not able to eat or drink due to her condition. She also has difficulty in communicating. Mrs Brown's daughter, Judith, has explained to the nursing staff that Mrs Brown, previous to her stroke, was active and meticulous in her personal hygiene and grooming. She believes that her mother will be very distressed due to not being able to attend to her appearance. It is clear to the admitting nurse that Judith is herself distressed by her mother's helplessness and by her not looking as she normally does. It is noted that Mrs Brown is perspiring, and that as she fell onto her bedroom floor during the night she has not had her usual morning bath. At this stage, three main problems can be identified regarding Mrs Brown's personal hygiene and grooming. These are concerned with Mrs Brown's inability to maintain skin and mouth hygiene due to her present illness and the emotional impact these factors may have on her sense of self and dignity.

NURSING PROBLEM 4.1

Problem: Mrs Brown is unable to maintain her skin hygiene needs due to impaired mobility and increased perspiration.

Goal: Mrs Brown's normal level of skin hygiene will be maintained.

Maintaining skin hygiene

A physical assessment of Mrs Brown's skin should be made while assisting her to meet her hygiene needs. The assessment should include (Penzer and Finch 2001):

- observing for skin changes (Colour: jaundice, bruising, pallor and inflammation.)
- skin integrity (Is the skin intact or are there lesions, sores or ulcers?)
- texture, moisture and heat (Use the back of the hand to assess the temperature of the skin.)
- hygiene (Is there evidence of neglect of grooming – strong or strange odours? Evidence of infestation – spots, scratching?).

A daily bed bath will be undertaken until Mrs Brown can be taken to the bathroom for a normal bath and, due to her increased perspiration, additional sponging will be administered as necessary.

The feeling of comfort that follows a well-executed bed bath should not be underestimated for its potential to lift the patient's morale and to induce feelings of wellbeing. A daily wash removes skin cell build-up and the bacteria that interact with perspiration to produce body odour. Bath time is a good opportunity for the nurse to give private, personal time to Mrs Brown, talking with her and encouraging her to express herself as best she can. This is also a good opportunity for the nurse to assess the state of the patient's skin and note the condition of pressure areas (see Chapter 5).

Intervention: the bed bath

Equipment

- Clean linen.
- Bowl of warm water (should be bowl for patient's personal use).
- Large bath towel, or small cotton blanket and smaller towel.
- Disposable wipes.
- Patient's wash cloth (should not be used for perineal area).
- Disposal bag.
- Patient's toiletries: soap or emollient, deodorant, cologne and talcum powder if used.

Procedure

- The nurse should explain that Mrs Brown is to be washed in bed and why, and reassured that as soon as possible she will be offered a normal bath.

- Care should be taken to ensure Mrs Brown's privacy by ensuring the bed is screened.
- Mrs Brown should be kept warm by ensuring that the room temperature is optimal, that there are no draughts and that she is covered at all times.
- The nurse should collect together and take to the bedside the equipment needed for total personal care.

TIP! The skin of older people such as Mrs Brown is subject to normal changes of ageing that result from reduced production of natural oils. This may make the skin dry and itchy. If soap is to be used it should be unperfumed and moisturized. It may be preferable to use emollients or aqueous cream to maintain the skin's normal function and to promote comfort (Penzer and Finch 2001).

- The bed is stripped down to the top sheet, and the patient made comfortable with pillows.

TIP! Ergonomically, it is preferable for two carers to assist the patient with a bed bath as this avoids hazardous manoeuvres of stretching over the patient for washing or moving the patient. Make sure that the bed is raised to a height that is safe for both carers. To prevent dripping water over the cleaned limb, wash, rinse and dry the limb furthest away from the water basin first, the nurse nearest the water passing the cloth/wipe to the second carer. If only one carer is involved she should consider moving from side to side of the bed.

- The patient is assisted to remove clothing, keeping the patient covered at all times with the top sheet.
- The bath sheet is laid over the top sheet, which is then slipped away from under the bath sheet and removed, leaving the patient covered by the bath sheet.
- The face is washed first. The patient should be asked how they normally clean their face (some people do not like soap or water on their face and prefer to use cleansing lotion). Many patients have a separate washcloth for face and body but patients should be advised that in the interests of infection control, disposable wipes would be used for the perineum and genitalia.

- The water should be changed whenever necessary but always after the genitals have been washed and before moving to the lower part of the body. Recommended practice is to have a separate basin available for washing the genital and perineal area and using disposable wipes.
- The body is then systematically washed, using soap or emollient, and then rinsing and drying from neck downwards towards the feet. One part of the body should be washed, rinsed and dried before moving to the next to prevent chilling and chafing. The suggested order is:
  - face and neck
  - chest
  - axilla and arm furthest away from water basin
  - axilla and arm nearest water basin
  - genitalia and perineum
  - change water
  - back
  - leg furthest away from water basin
  - leg nearest water basin
  - foot furthest away from water basin
  - foot nearest water basin.
- When washing the hands and feet note any abnormalities and record these. To enhance future mobility and comfort, it may be necessary to refer to a chiropodist if the patient's feet are in poor condition. Check that nails are clean and trim if required. It is necessary to check your Trust policies with respect to the clipping of nails, particularly those of diabetic patients. However, general principles are that fingernails and toenails should be softened by soaking in warm water prior to trimming. If dirty underneath, the nails should be cleaned with an orange stick whilst soaking in the water. After drying, the fingernails and/or toenails should be gently trimmed with nail scissors or clippers. Fingernails should be shaped following the curve of the fingertip and can be smoothed with an emery board. The toenails should be cut straight across.

TIP! **Enabling the patient to put hands and feet in basin to be washed is refreshing and achieves maximum comfort. The limbs should be supported and the basin steadied.**

● Toiletries such as anti-perspirant deodorants, talcum powder and cologne should be applied according to the patient's preferences. The use of toiletries helps to maintain skin freshness, and ensuring that a patient's preferences and normal habits are followed promotes the patient's dignity and sense of control.

TIP! **Protect the patient's face when using powders and sprays, as it is easy to affect the eyes and breathing with these when the patient is confined to bed. Talcum powder should be used lightly to prevent it 'pilling' into abrasive balls when patient's skin becomes damp with perspiration and should be avoided in the genital area if a patient has a urinary catheter in situ.**

Mrs Brown should be assisted into clean, 'light' (preferably cotton) nightclothes or other appropriate garment and her bed made up with clean linen as appropriate. The use of natural fibres such as cotton helps in the absorption of perspiration. Clean bed linen promotes the comfort and dignity of the patient.

Mrs Brown's hair should be brushed/combed into a style that is acceptable to herself and/or her daughter and comfortable to wear in bed.

Mrs Brown may not be able to adequately communicate her likes and dislikes and the nurse may need to consult with Judith to maintain or adapt Mrs Brown's grooming preferences. Maintaining as far as possible usual grooming routines promotes Mrs Brown's sense of self and individuality.

On completion of the procedure:

● If Mrs Brown is well enough to sit out in a chair, that is an ideal time to do her hair and teeth, since sitting up is a more normal position in which to attend to these areas.

● Mrs Brown's bed should be remade with fresh linen and she should be left comfortable with items she may require, such as call bell and tissues in reach.

● The basin should be cleaned, dried and stored according to Trust policy, disposable items placed in the appropriate receptacles, and soiled linen placed directly into the linen skip.

● Wash hands to prevent the spread of infection.

Record the procedure and any pertinent observations in the nursing records. This maintains necessary records and charts the patient's progress.

Mrs Brown should be sponged as necessary due to her increased perspiration, and garments changed if necessary.

Excessive perspiration on the skin is uncomfortable, can lead to chilling and disrupts the skin's protective functions. Remembering that the skin of older people is prone to dryness, over-frequent washing with soap should be avoided. However, for some patients where their medical condition may cause them to perspire freely, their comfort should be maintained by gentle sponging and drying of the skin (avoiding chilling) and providing fresh linen as necessary.

Mrs Brown should be offered handwashing facilities or the use of antiseptic hand wipes or rubs following the use of bedpans or other sanitary aids. Hand cleansing following the use of toileting aids is vital to the control of infection and maintains the normal routine of the patient.

As Mrs Brown recovers, she can gradually be encouraged to be more independent in washing and drying the parts of her body that she can reach herself during bathing in bed or in a chair at the side of the bed. This should be carefully managed, ensuring that Mrs Brown is acting within her capabilities and hygiene standards are maintained to her satisfaction.

As soon as Mrs Brown is able, she may be taken to the bathroom for a bath or shower and to have her hair washed. This return to a more normal routine will promote her dignity, recovery and rehabilitation.

Evaluation

Mrs Brown is clean and comfortable and either she or her family (if she is unable) expresses satisfaction with her personal hygiene.

Intervention: helping a patient have a bath or shower in the bathroom

Equipment

- Soap or emollient.
- Flannel or sponge.
- Disposable cloths if required for perineal care.

● Shampoo if required and brush and comb.
● Deodorant and other preferred toiletries.
● One small and one large towel.
● Toothbrush and paste.
● Clean nightclothes or other appropriate clothing.

Procedure

● Prepare the bathroom by ensuring that it is warm, the bath is clean and the necessary equipment is available, such as hoists, a shower chair, a shower trolley and non-slip mats.
● Gather washing equipment.
● Run the bath at a temperature that will be comfortable to the patient or arrange the bathroom for the patient to take a shower.

TIP! Serious burn accidents have occurred in relation to baths. Use a bath thermometer to ensure that the bath water is approximately 43°C and never more than 46°C (Potter and Perry 1997), taking great care with elderly patients who are more vulnerable to burn injury.

● The nurse should wear a clean plastic apron.
● Assist the patient to use the lavatory prior to commencing the bath or shower procedure.
● Assist the patient to the bathroom, ensure privacy can be maintained by locking the door or placing an 'engaged' notice on the door, and provide a screen to shield the bath area.

TIP! If the patient is able to bath himself unaided, ensure that a call button is available.

● Help the patient to undress, checking the skin condition and noting any bruising, rashes, lesions or other breaches of skin integrity.
● Recheck the water temperature of the bath or shower; if possible, the patient could use his hand to confirm the temperature is comfortable.
● Assist the patient into the bath, using a hoist if necessary, or into the shower, using a shower chair.

- Assist the patient to wash, encouraging him to do as much as possible for himself.
- If necessary, help the patient with hair washing, providing a cloth to protect the patient's eyes.

TIP! If washing the hair with the patient in the bath, use fresh water from the sink and either a jug or shower connection to rinse the hair. Check the water temperature is warm, not hot, to touch, before pouring it over the patient's head. Some elderly patients may find it difficult to lean their head back to prevent water flowing over their face as you rinse the hair, so provide a cloth to protect the eyes. Wrap the hair in a towel after washing, and make sure it is dried thoroughly to prevent the patient getting chilled. Style it appropriately after the bath; many clinical areas have rollers and hairdryers that can be used.

- In cases of patients suspected as having infestations of head lice, no form of treatment should be instigated until a confirmed diagnosis is gained. Local policies will direct interventions of 'wet combing' and specific insecticide treatment. Alternatively the 'Bug Busting' method may be implemented. 'Bug Busting' involves washing the hair with ordinary shampoo and fine-combing the damp, well-conditioned hair on repeated occasions. Recent studies have, however, suggested that insecticide lotion is more effective than 'Bug Busting' (NHS Direct Online 2001).
- Use the small towel to blot dry the hair and the face, and assist the patient out of the bath or shower.
- Cover the patient with the larger towel as soon as possible to prevent chilling and ensure privacy.
- Assist the patient to dry his body, apply preferred toiletries and dress.

TIP! Ensure crevices and creases are thoroughly dried. Obese patients or those with certain deformities may find it difficult to keep dry, particularly in the groin, under breasts, between the buttocks or in the umbilicus, and may develop skin lesions in these areas. If these occur, advice regarding appropriate dressings should be sought from senior staff, and all such lesions recorded in the nursing documentation.

● Facilitate teeth brushing/denture cleansing and assist arrangement of hair in preferred style.
● Male patients should be assisted to shave.

TIP! **Use a disposable or patient's own razor for wet shaving. If using a communal electric shaver, ensure it is thoroughly brushed out between patients and cleaned according to manufacturer's instructions.**

● Help the patient back to bed or chair and ensure he is comfortable. Return the patient's belongings to his locker.
● Clean the bath/shower according to Trust policy and leave it tidy.
● Record in the nursing notes the assessment of the patient's skin and the care that has been given. Accurate and complete records must be kept for all aspects of the patient's care. This adheres to the legal requirement of documenting and provides a baseline of data from which to monitor progress.

Evaluation

Has Mrs Brown had her personal hygiene needs met by having a bath or shower? Did she have sufficient energy for the procedure or was it too taxing? Did she manage to wash some parts of herself independently?

TIP! **Some patients are able to wash a little independently, but have not got the energy to have a full bath or shower. They may be assisted to have a wash either in bed or sitting out in the chair. The required equipment will be as for a bed bath, and the patient should be encouraged to wash as far as they are able. Clean hot water should be provided at appropriate intervals. The nurse can expect to assist washing the patient's back or feet or wherever is unreachable. It is helpful if the nurse is in the vicinity while the patient is washing in case the activity is too demanding, so that nursing support can be given quickly. Alternatively the patient may like to wash himself at the bathroom basin, as it is a more natural environment. Ensure privacy and dignity is maintained whichever location is chosen.**

NURSING PROBLEM 4.2

Problem: Mrs Brown is at risk of developing mouth infections and discomfort due to being unable to maintain her usual mouth hygiene or to eat and drink.

Goal: Mrs Brown's mouth will remain clean, moist and free from infection.

Oral hygiene

Mouth hygiene is an essential aspect of care for the dependent patient, and the nurse/carer must be able to assist patients to achieve an acceptable level of oral hygiene. Assistance with oral hygiene will be needed for patients with:

- limited mobility
- debilitating pain or movement restrictions
- altered consciousness levels
- cognitive problems, such as confusion in older people
- eating or drinking difficulties, resulting in the loss of the natural cleansing actions of saliva and potential dehydration
- breathlessness, due to loss of fluid from the respiratory tract
- compromised immune systems leading to increased risk of infection
- radiotherapy treatments to the head and neck
- oxygen therapy, which has drying effects on the oral mucosa.

Many people in the United Kingdom do not receive regular dental care and nurses may encounter hospital patients with problems with their teeth and gums or whose dentures no longer fit and/or are in poor condition (Evans 2001). Assessment of the mouth is therefore an important preliminary step in mouth care. Effective oral hygiene helps to prevent infection, distress and discomfort, and, in the case of patients such as Mrs Brown who may require speech therapy, it is a vital component of rehabilitation.

Patients who have natural teeth must be enabled to brush and irrigate their teeth. Brushing removes food particles, loosens plaque and stimulates blood flow to the gums. For patients who normally wear dentures, it is essential that they are enabled to wear them whenever possible. This promotes dignity and comfortable eating and maintains the shape of the mouth. However, it is not possible for some patients to wear their dentures, for example, if they are unconscious. Patients such as Mrs Brown will require a specialized assessment to determine when it becomes safe for her to wear her dentures.

Intervention: oral hygiene

Assess Mrs Brown's needs with respect to mouth care. Assessment to obtain initial information regarding the patient's oral health is necessary to provide baseline information and to assist the evaluation of mouth care interventions.

The following are indicators of a healthy mouth (Evans 2001):

● pink moist tongue, oral mucosa and gums
● teeth/dentures clean and free of debris
● well-fitting dentures
● adequate salivation
● smooth and moist lips
● no difficulties with eating and drinking.

Undertake mouth care on a regular basis according to the patient's needs.

Cleaning the teeth or mouth after every meal will refresh patients' mouths but toothpaste should not be used too frequently (see below). Patients with dry mouths may appreciate opportunities to rinse their mouths with diluted mouthwash or fresh water several times a day between meals.

Equipment

● Disposable cup.
● Small torch.
● Mouthwash solution made up with fresh water.
● Receiver or small bowl.
● Protective towel.
● Tissues.

- Foam sticks.
- Wooden spatula.
- Small-headed soft toothbrush.
- Toothpaste.
- Disposable gloves.
- Denture pot and denture cleaning agent and brush.

Procedure

- The nurse should explain to Mrs Brown that her mouth is to be examined and cleaned, to reassure her and gain her consent and cooperation.
- The nurse should wash her hands and then prepare the solutions; disposable gloves should be worn to undertake the procedure and the protective towel placed over Mrs Brown's chest. This prevents cross-infection and avoids spillage on Mrs Brown's gown and linen.
- If Mrs Brown is wearing dentures, they should be removed, rinsed and placed in a denture pot with cleansing solution. If assessment indicates that it is not yet safe for Mrs Brown to wear her dentures, they should be cleaned and stored in a named container. This ensures safe-keeping of Mrs Brown's property and maintains hygiene of dentures.

TIP! **Removing dentures is easier if a tissue or gauze swab is used to hold them with.**

- The nurse/carer should inspect Mrs Brown's mouth, using the wooden spatula to hold the tongue down gently. Care should be taken not to place the spatula too far back on the tongue as this may induce the gag reflex and make Mrs Brown frightened and uncomfortable.
- Mrs Brown's mouth should be pink and moist. The condition of her mouth should be noted and any bleeding areas or ulcers should be reported to the nurse in charge of her care. This ensures that the baseline condition of the mouth is established.
- The small-headed soft toothbrush and toothpaste should be used to gently brush any natural teeth Mrs Brown may have, and her gums and tongue (Turner 1996), again taking care not to induce the gag reflex.

TIP! **A child's or baby's toothbrush is an ideal size to use if the patient cannot manipulate the toothbrush himself as it is less likely to cause trauma to the gums and palate.**

- Inner and outer aspects of any teeth should be cleaned with the soft toothbrush, brushing away from the gums. Gums and tongue should be brushed very gently to prevent any injury. Foam sticks are soft and can be used frequently to refresh the mouth, but do not remove plaque (Burglass 1995; Moore 1995).
- Toothpaste is drying and can burn vulnerable gums. It should be carefully rinsed away. Where patients are able to rinse out their mouths, offer the disposable cup containing fresh water or mouthwash. Where patients are unable to rinse out their mouths themselves, use a rinsed toothbrush and swab the mouth with a foam stick. Use the tissues to wipe the mouth.

TIP! **When cleaning an unconscious patient's teeth, use the oral suction equipment and Yankuer sucker to aspirate all fluid whilst rinsing the teeth to prevent it from trickling down the patient's throat and causing them to cough or gag (see Chapter 8).**

- Vaseline or soft paraffin can be applied to the lips with a gauze swab to keep lips moist and soft.
- Mrs Brown's dentures should be thoroughly cleaned with denture-cleansing products and brush and replaced if appropriate or stored in a named container/denture pot.
- All solutions should be discarded and the equipment cleaned and replaced.
- Mrs Brown should be made comfortable.
- The nurse/carer should wash her hands.

Evaluation

Does Mrs Brown have a moist, clean mouth and gums? Is her mouth free from infection?

NURSING PROBLEM 4.3

Problem: Mrs Brown may be distressed and her dignity compromised by not being able to maintain her normal grooming habits.

Goal: Mrs Brown will have her normal grooming habits met.

Personal dressing and grooming

Mrs Brown's condition will have resulted in an alteration in her body image. How a person feels about himself is directly related to how the body is perceived by that person (Salter 1988). Disturbances in body image can, therefore, be distressing. An attempt to maintain Mrs Brown's usual grooming habits and to promote her presentation as attractively as possible positively influences her sense of self and gives her some control over her personal environment

Maintain Mrs Brown's privacy at all times when undertaking personal care. Ensure Mrs Brown's privacy is protected, thus demonstrating respect to her as a person and assisting her to maintain dignity and control over her personal environment.

Ensure that Mrs Brown's own toiletries are available for use when attending to her hygiene needs.

TIP! **Advise Mrs Brown's daughter to provide toiletries that Mrs Brown prefers but to select those with scents that are light and fresh. Heavy perfumes can seem unpleasant to ill people. Think carefully about whether it is advisable for Mrs Brown to use her favourite scents. She may find this comforting but she may also later come to associate that scent with the unpleasant experience of being ill.**

Encourage Judith to help her mother to apply moisturizer and make-up prior to visitors if she wears it as this assists both Mrs Brown and her family to maintain her personal image.

Ensure that Mrs Brown's hair is styled in her preferred manner, as guided by herself or her daughter. She may like to visit the hospital hairdresser when she is feeling better, or be helped to wash and style her hair when her medical condition allows.

Encourage Judith to provide attractive nightwear or other garments for Mrs Brown to wear; she may require some advice about appropriate garments. For example, if Mrs Brown is incontinent, clothing that is easily laundered will be necessary, and items that are easy for Mrs Brown to put on and off should be provided.

It will be essential for Judith to bring in well-fitting house shoes or slippers that have non-slip soles and that support Mrs Brown's feet so that as she begins to mobilize her safety needs can be met. Further advice as to suitable footwear can be obtained from the physiotherapist.

Nightclothes may not always be appropriate for daywear, especially for long-stay patients who may need to attend therapy sessions in the hospital. Daywear should be easy to put on, especially if there is paralysis in upper or lower limbs. It is good practice to insert the affected limb first into clothes and remove it last as the other non-paralysed limb is more flexible. Aids to assist dressing such as button or bra hooks may be required, and the occupational therapist will assist in assessing Mrs Brown's additional dressing needs.

Ensure that, if appropriate and safe, Mrs Brown is wearing her dentures during the day.

Evaluation

Is Mrs Brown well-presented in her own clothes? If Mrs Brown is able to express a preference, is she satisfied with her personal grooming and presentation? Is her daughter?

Further reading

Burglass EA (1995) Oral hygiene. British Journal of Nursing 4(9): 516–19.

Evans G (2001) A rationale for oral care. Nursing Standard 15(43): 33–36.

Moore J (1995) Assessment of nurse-administered hygiene. Nursing Times 91(9): 40–41.

NHS Direct Online (2001) http://www.healthcareguide.nhsdirect.nhs.uk/conditions/lice/lice.stm (accessed 26/09/01).

Penzer R, Finch M (2001) Promoting healthy skin on older people. Nursing Standard 15(34): 46–52.

Potter AP, Perry AG (eds) (1997) Fundamentals of Nursing: Concepts, Process and Practice, 4th edn. St Louis: Mosby.
Salter M (ed.) (1988) Altered Body Image: The Nurse's Role. London: Wiley.
Turner G (1996) Oral care. Nursing Standard 10(28): 51–54.

CHAPTER 5

Preventing the complications of bed-rest

Frances Gordon

Aims and learning outcomes

This chapter considers the complications that can arise as a result of restricted mobility associated with bed-rest and how the risk of these complications may be prevented or reduced. By the end of this chapter you will be able to:

- recognize the danger of complications arising from bed-rest
- anticipate when a patient may be at risk of developing complications due to bed-rest
- understand the necessity of undertaking a thorough assessment of the patient
- implement measures that reduce the risk to the patient with respect to preventing deep vein thrombosis, chest infection and pressure ulcers.

The hazards of immobility

The human body is designed to be active and mobile. However, many of our patients or clients have difficulty with being mobile due to many reasons. These may include factors associated with genetic or acquired handicap; trauma; degenerative illnesses; the post-operative recovery period; and acute illnesses. Immobility can carry serious complications and active interventions are required to reduce the risk of these complications occurring. Among the hazards of immobility are the following:

- an increased incidence of deep vein thrombosis
- pulmonary embolism
- chest infection
- loss of skin integrity including decubitus ulcers (pressure sores)
- constipation
- urinary calculi
- urinary infection
- the development of atrophy, weakness of the muscles and osteoporosis that further increases the risk of renal calculi (Long et al. 1995).

These complications are well recognized, and patients are therefore encouraged to mobilize as soon as possible following surgery, childbirth or incapacitating illness. However, despite the early mobilization strategies of current healthcare, some patients still have their mobility compromised and so carry the potential to develop one or more of the complications of limited mobility. The nurse must actively work towards preventing these complications as far as possible. The complications that will be elaborated upon in this chapter are deep vein thrombosis and pulmonary embolism, chest infection and decubitus ulcers. The interventions aimed at minimizing the risk of these problems occurring will be individualized according to the needs of the patient, although the principles of care remain similar in each case. Complications arising from problems of immobility can appear very rapidly and it is important to remain focused on their prevention from the onset of the period of the reduced mobility.

Patient history

A typical patient who would require care related to the prevention of these complications is Mr Patel. Mr Patel is 60 years old and a retired accountant. He has been admitted to hospital due to a sudden collapse and is to have investigations. Mr Patel is a smoker but does not drink alcohol. Until this incident he has been in what he describes as 'good health' but since his collapse feels weak and exhausted. He will be assisted to sit out of bed and to begin mobilizing quite soon after his admission to hospital but, nevertheless, his mobility will be compromised for some days. The nurse will explain to Mr Patel that he will be asked to engage in certain activities in order to prevent complications arising from his anticipated short-term reduction in mobility. Three potential problems that face Mr Patel will be discussed and ways to minimize the risks will be considered.

Deep vein thrombosis

The first problem concerns Mr Patel's risk of developing a deep vein thrombosis and subsequent pulmonary embolism due to restricted mobility. Deep vein thrombosis is the formation of a clot (thrombus) in the deep veins of the leg due to venous stasis, damage to vein wall or the blood tending to clot more readily than normal (Long et al. 1995). Pulmonary embolism, a severe and life-threatening occurrence, can follow a deep vein thrombosis when a particle of the thrombus breaks away and travels in the blood stream to the lungs. Mr Patel is also at increased risk of deep vein thrombosis because he smokes. Other risk factors are obesity; pregnancy; the effects of surgical operations, particularly those of the pelvis or abdomen; and in orthopaedic patients who have mobility problems, fractures of the hips or spinal injury. There is a small increased risk among women who use oral contraception (Guillebaud 2000) and even smaller increased risk among women using hormone replacement therapy (Lindsay 1998).

NURSING PROBLEM 5.1

Problem: Mr Patel is at risk of developing a deep vein thrombosis and subsequent pulmonary embolism due to restricted mobility.
Goal: Mr Patel will not develop these complications.

Intervention: preventing deep vein thrombosis

The nurse should teach Mr Patel foot, leg and breathing exercises to practise whilst he is in bed. Trusting Mr Patel to undertake the exercises will enable him to feel in some control over his health and recovery.

Mr Patel should be reminded and encouraged to undertake his foot, leg and breathing exercises every hour. Frequent leg exercises are important to prevent the stasis of blood in the lower limbs, and deep breathing assists venous return to the heart.

Exercises

A full cycle of active exercises should be undertaken by the patient at least every hour to maintain the circulation:

- the leg muscles should be tightened and relaxed 10 times to 'pump' blood along veins
- the toes should be flexed and extended 10 times
- the foot should be flexed and extended at the ankle 10 times
- the knee should be flexed and extended 10 times
- the hip should be flexed and extended 10 times bringing the knee towards the chest
- the patient should take 10 deep breaths.

Mr Patel should be encouraged not to cross his legs, have them flexed for long periods or sit or lie with pressure under the calves, for example, by placing a pillow beneath the calves. These activities promote venous stasis and so predispose thrombus formation by exerting direct pressure on the leg veins.

Compression stockings

Mr Patel should be fitted with graduated compression stockings (thrombo-embolic deterrent – TED – stockings). It has been shown that the use of graduated compression stockings is effective in preventing deep vein thrombosis in hospital patients (Amarigiri and Lees 1999). The use of these stockings may be contraindicated in some patients with peripheral vascular disease or diabetic neuropathy (Campbell 2001). The correct size of stockings must be ascertained by taking accurate measurements with a tape measure, according to the manufacturer's instructions.

Applying graduated compression stockings

- The correct size of stockings should be taken to the patient's bedside.
- Privacy should be ensured for the patient by screening the bed.
- A non-threatening and supportive explanation of why the stockings are necessary should be given to the patient.

- Stockings should be measured and fitted according to the manufacturer's instructions.
- Stockings should be wrinkle-free.
- The patient should be advised not to partially roll down the stocking as this can impede circulation.
- Stockings should be removed and replaced daily for hygiene needs and to check condition of the skin.
- Observations of skin colour, skin integrity and perfusion should be recorded.

TIP! **A light dusting of talcum powder helps in the application of the compression stockings by reducing friction.**

Hydration

Mr Patel should be adequately hydrated by offering fluids hourly (see Chapter 7), since dehydration increases the risk of formation of deep vein thrombosis.

Anti-coagulants

Mr Patel should receive anti-coagulant prophylaxis as prescribed. This is usually in the form of prophylactic subcutaneous injections of heparin, which prevents the formation of blood clots and may be prescribed for predisposed or high-risk patients.

Observations

Mr Patel should be monitored for signs of the development of deep vein thrombosis and pulmonary embolism every x hours. Careful monitoring should detect complications early, and enable speedy instigation of treatment. Thrombus formation is often a 'silent' process. However, pain or tenderness in the calf, swelling and change in temperature may indicate a deep vein thrombosis, and the affected calf may appear paler than the other. Sudden difficulty in breathing and chest pain must be immediately reported as this could signify the medical emergency of pulmonary embolism.

The following checklist summarizes what should be monitored:

- pyrexia
- pain in the calf

- swelling of the calf (measure both legs with a tape measure for comparison)
- temperature of the leg (the affected calf may appear pale and cold if a calf vein is occluded and warm if a more superficial vein is inflamed)
- chest pain and/or difficulty in breathing.

Evaluation

Mr Patel remains free from the development of deep vein thrombosis and pulmonary embolism.

Chest infection

The second problem is associated with Mr Patel being at increased risk of developing a chest infection due to the restrictions on his mobility (caused by his illness and also his smoking habit). Chest infection can occur in people with restricted mobility because proper ventilation and drainage of respiratory secretions are inadequate, and the secretions pool and become a focus for infection. The patient may develop what is termed hypostatic pneumonia, a serious – and in some patients life-threatening – chest infection. These risks are increased among people who smoke. Patients who have undergone surgical operations are also at additional risk due to several factors: anaesthetic gases may irritate the lungs; the drugs used during and after surgery may reduce the patient's ability to breathe deeply or cough; and post-operative pain may make the patient unwilling or fearful to cough.

NURSING PROBLEM 5.2

Problem: Mr Patel is at increased risk of developing a chest infection due to restricted mobility and his smoking habit.

Goal: Mr Patel will remain free from chest infection.

Intervention: preventing chest infection

The nurse should teach Mr Patel deep breathing exercises (see Long et al. 1995) and encourage him to do them hourly.

Teaching Mr Patel to undertake the exercises will enable him to feel in some control over his health and recovery. Deep breathing exercises enable the chest to expand fully and promote the movement of respiratory secretions.

Breathing exercises

- Ensure patient's privacy.
- Provide sputum pot, tissues and mouthwash.
- The patient should sit upright with knees flexed.
- Place a hand lightly on the abdomen.
- Breathe in slowly through the nose until abdomen is felt to rise.
- Hold breath for 5 seconds.
- Exhale through pursed lips slowly.
- Repeat 7 times.

Mr Patel should be encouraged to cough and expectorate any sputum – sputum pot, tissues and mouthwash should be provided. Coughing encourages the movement of secretions in the chest to prevent pooling. Expectoration clears the chest and collection of sputum in pot allows for inspection and monitoring for signs of infection. Discoloured, blood stained and/or malodorous sputum should be reported to the nurse in charge and sent for laboratory investigation (see Chapter 8).

TIP! Some patients may be fearful or unwilling to cough because of pain – particularly following abdominal surgery or chest trauma/surgery. Ensure that the patient has been given adequate analgesia approximately 30 minutes prior to breathing and coughing exercises, and provide a soft pillow for the patient to use to splint his abdomen during coughing.

Cessation of smoking

The nurse should remind Mr Patel of the importance of not smoking in order to prevent the development of a chest infection and other complications whilst his mobility is restricted.

Smoking increases the risk of chest infection. A sensitive approach needs to be taken towards patients to encourage them to abstain from smoking during hospitalization and the period of acute illness. Supportive acknowledgement of the patient's smoking needs and careful explanations of why smoking will increase the risk of acute complications during illness empowers the patient to make positive decisions regarding his health. The following practical suggestions may assist the patient: exploring the triggers for smoking; implementing distraction activities such as reading, radio and television; and keeping a diary of feelings surrounding smoking resulting in success in overcoming the desire to smoke. Later in the recovery period, when Mr Patel is mobile again, not visiting any smoking areas may help him to avoid smoking. Prior to discharge, patients can be encouraged to consider longer-term smoking cessation by providing health promotion information and advice regarding access to further support, such as smoking cessation sessions at their local primary health care clinic.

Observations

Monitor Mr Patel's vital signs for evidence of infection. This ensures that signs of infection will be detected: report elevation in temperature, pulse and respiratory rate (see Chapter 2).

Hydration

Mr Patel should be adequately hydrated. Adequate hydration reduces the risk of sputum becoming tenacious and difficult to expectorate (see Chapter 8).

Evaluation

Mr Patel will be discharged from hospital without having developed a chest infection.

Pressure ulcers

The third problem arises from Mr Patel's potential to develop decubitus ulcers due to his restricted mobility. Pressure ulcers, also called decubitus ulcers or pressure sores, are localized areas of tissue damage resulting from direct pressure – for example, the weight of the patient's body lying in one position on the bed surface – or from shearing forces that cause mechanical damage between skin and bone and result in tissue ischaemia (Pedley 1999). Pressure ulcers usually occur over bony prominences such as the sacrum, knees and hips (NHS Centre for Reviews and Dissemination 1995). Among the patients at high risk for developing pressure ulcers are the following:

- those prone to remaining in one position due to mobility difficulties, pain, breathlessness, diminished sensation or cognitive problems
- those with impaired skin condition due to, for example, oedema or excessive skin dryness, or where there is risk of skin irritation and maceration as with continence problems
- those who are malnourished or who have hydration problems
- those with either low or high body mass index (see Chapter 9)
- those with certain medical conditions such as diabetes
- those taking medication that affects the skin, for example, steroids.

NURSING PROBLEM 5.3

Problem: Mr Patel is at risk of developing pressure ulcers (sores) due to restricted mobility.

Goal: Mr Patel's pressure areas will remain intact.

Intervention: reducing the risks of pressure ulcers

Risk assessment

The first procedure is to assess Mr Patel's risk of developing a pressure sore. Assessing a patient's risk of developing a pressure sore is a complex and lengthy exercise. Most units make this task more manageable by utilizing a risk assessment scale. Risk assessment scales have been developed to help the nurse identify those patients who are most likely to develop tissue impairment (Gould 2001). There are various scales available; all have their strengths and weaknesses. The general principles of pressure sore risk assessment scales are that they identify risk factors of:

- mobility
- nutritional status
- continence problems
- the patient's general physical condition.

Probably the most common scale in use in the UK is the Waterlow Scale; it is arguably the most comprehensive and covers other factors such as age, weight, disease process and medication, all of which, as described above, may predispose the patient to developing pressure sores (Gould 2001). The locally preferred scale should be used in the clinical area, but be aware that other scales are available, and more refined examples may be already available or be developed over time. The assessment of a patient's pressure sore risk enables identification of the level and types of interventions required for an individual. It is important, however, not to rely on risk assessment scales alone – the nurse's clinical judgement should also be employed.

Maintaining mobility

Explain to Mr Patel the importance of moving around the bed as much as possible. Assist Mr Patel to change position to relieve pressure on pressure areas every two hours using recommended manual handling techniques. Relief of pressure is essential to prevent tissue damage, and appropriate manual handling techniques are essential to prevent friction and shear injury.

Encouraging the patient to avoid remaining in one position for long periods helps to prevent pressure on the bony prominences. However, Mr Patel should be warned about movements that may involve a shearing action on the bed surface. Shearing movements involve friction, such as dragging the skin over the bed surface rather than lifting his skin above the surface of the bed or chair before moving, or using a sliding sheet when helping Mr Patel change position. Pressure sores can be prevented by good bed-making, which smooths creases in bed linen or the patient's garments. Damp sheets resulting from perspiration or urine should be changed promptly. Make sure that crumbs or other small objects (including catheters or drainage tubes) do not get trapped against the patient's skin and cause pressure. Also, make sure that the top covers are not too tight and restricting to the patient's movements.

TIP! Advise Mr Patel to use television or radio timings as reminders for him to change his position on a regular basis.

Skin inspection

Inspect the skin at each position change and record condition of pressure areas. Early detection of skin changes that may indicate pressure problems is essential. These include fixed red marks that do not fade (erythema): blanching if gentle pressure is applied indicates that circulation is still intact; however, if the area of redness does not blanch, disruption to the microcirculation is evident. Erythema is more difficult to detect on darker skins such as Mr Patel's, so attention should be paid to swelling, change in skin temperature, and discomfort. It is important that an accurate record of the patient's skin condition is maintained. This ensures that interventions are appropriately implemented according to the patient's condition.

Use of pressure-relieving aids

Pressure-relieving aids such as specialized mattresses or beds may be indicated in high-risk patients with very restricted mobility. Furniture such as chairs should be carefully chosen to ensure that the patient is able to rise from them easily. If able, Mr Patel should be encouraged to relieve pressure by standing or taking short walks or to make frequent small movements when sitting for longer periods. It may also be appropriate to use gel cushions in the patient's chair as a means of preventing excessive pressure. Careful use of pillows can help avoid pressure on heels and elbows but care must be taken not to place pillows under patients' calves.

TIP! **When using appliances such as commodes or bedpans assist patients from them promptly as hard edges can damage the skin.**

Nutrition

Ensure that Mr Patel's nutritional status is adequate and that he remains hydrated. Poor nutrition and inadequate hydration are factors that increase the risk of pressure ulcer formation (see Chapter 9).

Skin hygiene

Ensure that Mr Patel's skin hygiene is maintained to a high standard. Skin breakdown is more likely in patients who are incontinent, due to the presence of moisture-containing bacteria that can cause skin maceration. The maintenance of skin hygiene is therefore very important in the prevention of pressure ulcers, but care must be taken not to cause over-drying of the skin by the use of frequent soap application. Emollients should be considered instead of soap for cleaning (see Chapter 4), and also the use of barrier creams to protect the skin from exposure to urine and faeces.

Evaluation

Mr Patel will be discharged from hospital with his skin free from the development of pressure ulcers.

Further reading

Long BC, Phipps WJ, Cassmeyer VL (1995) Adult Nursing: A Nursing Process Approach. London: Mosby.

NHS Centre for Reviews and Dissemination (1995) The Prevention and Treatment of Pressure Sores. York: NHS CRD.

Caring for patients who need nursing support

CHAPTER 6

Drug administration

Barbara Workman

Aims and learning outcomes

This chapter describes the role of the nurse when administering medications, and outlines the principles of safe administration of medication by the commonest routes. By the end of this chapter you will be able to do the following:

- state and apply the five Rights (5 Rs) of safe drug administration
- outline the A–F points for safe practice
- calculate a common drug dose
- undertake safe administration of oral, rectal, parenteral and eye medications under supervision.

Administering medication

The administration of medications is controlled by three Acts of Parliament – the Medicines Act (1968), the Misuse of Drugs Act (1971) and the Poisons Act (1972) – and a Statutory Instrument – the Misuse of Drugs Regulations (1985). These provide the framework within which medicines are stored, transported, prescribed, recorded, dispensed and administered. The British National Formulary (BNF) provides a summary of the key legal issues for health care practitioners, which is beyond the scope of this chapter but can be referred to for further guidance. You should also familiarize yourself with local policies and guidelines, which should be available in your workplace for reference.

Advances in treatment and drug therapy progress rapidly in nursing and medicine, and as professional research and knowledge expands so must your repertoire of knowledge, to underpin safe practice. The guidelines for safe practice are outlined in this chapter but it is the responsibility of individual practitioners check the product information of each drug during its administration, in order to verify the dose, route, time, method of administration and contraindications. When administering the drug you must ensure that proper procedures have been followed.

Administering drugs by different routes and for various purposes is a common activity in nursing. The UKCC Guidelines for the Administration of Medicines emphasize that 'in administering any medication, or assisting or overseeing any self administration of medication, you must exercise your professional judgement and apply your knowledge and skill in the given situation' (2000: 4). This means that you should have:

● knowledge of the drug
● know its effects and potential side effects
● know the patient's condition
● assess the suitability for that medication at that given time.

The five Rights (5 Rs) of drug administration

The responsibility for administering medication safely is one which nurses take seriously, and to assist in this procedure the five Rights (5 Rs) of drug administration have been devised:

● Right patient
● Right drug
● Right dose
● Right time
● Right route.

Right patient

Check the identity of the patient with his identification band, using hospital number or date of birth as additional verification. If patients are long-stay residents, identification may be by photograph, rather than an impersonal name band (Williams 1996). In the home setting you should satisfy yourself that you have identified the right patient for medication by asking them their full name or date of birth to verify against the prescription.

Right drug

Drug names can be complex, and have similarities between names. Check for clearly written prescriptions, matching the name on the medication container. In hospital, drugs are prescribed by their generic names, and patients may be confused and think that they are having a new medication. If in doubt, consult the BNF for the generic and trade name of the drug.

Check three times during the procedure:

● when you take the drug from the cupboard or trolley
● before you pour it into the medication receiver, matching it to the drug name on the prescription sheet
● as you return it to the cupboard or trolley.

Right dose

This should be clearly written on the prescription sheet. If the dose is very small, then micrograms should be written out in full (BNF). Calculate the dose carefully (page 99) and check to see if there is a drug with the same name but dispensed in different strengths.

TIP! **If you need to calculate the dose, make sure you know what the usual dose is likely to be so that if your calculations result in an unusual number, like six tablets rather than two, you are alerted to check it again, preferably with another person.**

Right time

Most drugs are designed to be given with an interval of several hours apart to provide a consistent therapeutic blood level. If given haphazardly, then the medication will be less effective or may cause the patient to develop unwanted side effects. Therefore, it is essential to give doses at prescribed intervals and to record the actual time of administration.

Right route

Medications are given licences for specific routes of administration. It is possible to give medication by the wrong route, for example, an intramuscular injection may be given intravenously if sited in the wrong place.

The A–F of safe practice

To ensure safe administration, some other principles can be considered. These are listed below as the A–F of safe practice:

- Accurate prescription
- Best information
- Correct dispensing
- Deliberation before administration
- Effective systems
- Fail-safe policies.

Accurate prescription

Prescription sheets should be clearly written, and should include the patient's name and hospital number, weight and allergies – or state 'no allergies known'. It should include the doctor's signature, and the date of commencement or discontinuation of medication. The generic name of the prescribed drug should be used. Abbreviations should not be used for micrograms or nanograms. Doses should be in specific metric measures rather than number of tablets, for example, *paracetamol 1 g* rather than *paracetamol 2 tabs*. Following administration, all documentation should be completed accurately and legibly, and using the accepted local abbreviations, for example if the patient is 'nil by mouth' and cannot take his medicine, then that should be recorded on the prescription sheet.

TIP! **If you withhold a drug for any reason, make sure that the medical staff know. It may need to be given by another route, or its suitability for that patient may need to be reviewed.**

Best information

Your patient has a right to ask you about his medication, and you should be able to explain what the medication is for. The patient may not wish to take his medication without knowing how it may affect him. A nurse's role is to teach the patient about his medications:

- how and when to take them
- recognizable effects and side effects
- when, if ever, to stop the treatment.

Understanding medication is more likely to help your patient follow his treatment.

When you are administering the medication you should be able to easily access drug information in the clinical area, such as the British National Formulary (BNF) or Data Compendium sheets. If you are unfamiliar with the drug, it is good nursing practice not to administer the drug until you have familiarized yourself with the expected effects and side effects and requisite patient monitoring during the course of treatment. Always consult the pharmacist if you have any uncertainties about a drug.

Correct dispensing

Pharmacists dispense many medications daily and may occasionally make errors. The nurse should ensure that the dispensed drug is correct against the prescribed drug. This is particularly necessary when the drug has been prepared in the pharmacy and is ready for administration without further preparation in the clinical area. The dose, labelling and prescription should be checked for any peculiarities before administration. If you are unfamiliar with the dose or drug do not assume that it is right. Confirm the dose rather than cause a severe error.

Deliberation before administration

It is easy to be sidetracked and distracted from tasks in a busy clinical area where there are many interruptions. Medication errors may result because such distractions can prevent busy nurses from recognizing warning signals during the procedure. It is important that drugs are prepared in a quiet location if possible, and that the task is completed before another begun. It is also important that nurses should feel able to stop and think, to check when uncertain and to gather additional information to clarify any questions they may have about the drugs that are being prepared (Colleran Cook 1999).

Effective systems

Studies have demonstrated that if systems and procedures are not followed, there is an increased likelihood of medication errors (O'Shea 1999). A counter check against error can be provided by the use of a structured routine, such as this:

- always use the prescription chart, and do not administer from memory
- always check patient identification – even when the patient is well known
- never administer something you did not witness being prepared
- do not leave drugs on lockers to be taken later
- do not return an unused dose to a stock bottle
- never leave an open drug cupboard or trolley unattended.

Such systems should alert you to danger signals that may lead to an error, thereby adding security to the proceedings.

Fail-safe policies

The Trust that you work for should have clear policies concerning the mechanisms, supervision and training for drug administration, and for reporting 'near misses'. These should be followed not only to prevent error and subsequent litigation but also because such policies encourage good practice. However, there may be changes in knowledge and clinical practice that become accepted practice within the Trust, but are not recorded immediately within Policies (Colleran Cook 1999). You may need to ensure that your Manager is aware of these changes in practice to ensure that the local Policies reflect actual current practice. For example, to reduce errors and spread the workload, your unit may decide that night staff will not give drugs in the morning but wait for the day staff to do it. Local policy may need to take that change into account so that nursing and medical staff are all aware of it.

TIP! To reduce potential errors you should only administer drugs to your group of patients, so that you are familiar with their particular needs. Also, consider the timing of doses. If a patient needs to take some medication before and some after his meal, don't be tempted to give it to him all at once, relying on him to remember to take them after eating. He may leave the medicine on his locker and either forget it or another patient may take it by mistake. It takes longer to sort out mistakes than to go to your patient twice!

Calculating drug dosages

It is important in drug calculations to be able to understand the values of the drug doses and their relationship to one another.

The measurement of weight for drugs is expressed in grams (g), milligrams (mg) and micrograms (mcg). Patients are weighed in kilograms (kg). The measurement of fluid volumes is usually expressed in litres (l) or millilitres (ml).

- 1 kilogram = 1 000 grams
- 1 gram = 1 000 milligrams
- 1 milligram = 1 000 micrograms
- 1 litre = 1 000 millilitres

Converting measurements

To change kilograms to grams, *multiply* by 1 000:
e.g. 5 kg × 1 000 = 5 000 g

To change grams to milligrams, *multiply* by 1 000:
e.g. 5 g × 1 000 = 5 000 mg

To change milligrams to micrograms, *multiply* by 1 000:
e.g. 0.625 mg × 1 000 = 625 micrograms

To change milligrams to grams, *divide* by 1 000:
e.g. 500 mg ÷ 1 000 = 0.5 g

To change micrograms to milligrams, *divide* by 1 000:
e.g. 250 mcg ÷ 1 000 = 0.25 mg

Calculating drug dosages

To calculate drug dosages the following formula may be used:

$$\frac{\text{What you want}}{\text{What you've got}} \times \text{total volume} = \text{dose required}$$

Example: a prescription requires 30 mg of a drug that is dispensed as 60 mg in 5 ml

$$\frac{\text{What you want: 30 mg}}{\text{What you've got: 60 mg}} \times \text{total volume: 5 ml} = \frac{30}{60} \times 5 = 2.5 \text{ ml required}$$

It is important to ensure that the units are consistent in the calculation, i.e. either all milligrams or all micrograms. If the numbers are not all converted to the same units, drug errors up to 1 000 times too big or too small may occur.

Example: a patient is prescribed Nifedipine 0.06 g. Tablets of Nifedipine are 20 mg strength. How many should be given?

$$\frac{\text{What you want: 0.06 g}}{\text{What you've got: 20 mg}} \times \text{volume: 1 tablet} = \text{dose required}$$

First the decimal 0.06 g must be converted into a whole number, consistent with the drug as dispensed:

0.06 g × 1 000 = 60 mg

The formula can then be used:

$$\frac{60 \text{ mg}}{20 \text{ mg}} \times 1 = 3 \text{ tablets}$$

NURSING PROBLEM 6.1

Patient history: Mr Jenkins has just been admitted with worsening of Parkinson's disease. He has come in to have his medication reviewed. He can be very stiff, shaky and slow at times, especially when he has to pick up his pills.

Problem: Mr Jenkins requires assistance with his oral medication at times.

Goal: Mr Jenkins will be assisted to take his oral medication when necessary.

Oral medication

The oral route is the safest, most convenient and least expensive route for medication delivery. Oral drugs are available in many forms of tablets, capsules or granules, or liquids such as syrups, or suspensions. Most are suitable to be swallowed without further preparation, but some may need dissolving or mixing before consumption. If patients cannot swallow their medication because it is in an inappropriate preparation, such as a large tablet, advice from the pharmacist should be sought to see if an alternative preparation is available.

Planning

If several patients are to receive their medications at a set time, it is an acceptable practice to use a trolley stocked with all the equipment required (Williams 1996). Ideally this should be the group of patients that you are currently caring for.

This equipment should include:

- stock and specific personal prescription drugs – ensure adequate supplies, within expiry date
- medicine pots – to dispense individual medication
- disposable cups – to provide a drink to assist easy swallowing of medication, or to dissolve tablets if necessary
- water jug, freshly filled, to ensure water is easily available
- straws – some patients find it easier to take unpalatable medicine through a straw, and a straw may help a patient with swallowing difficulties to wash tablets down more easily
- teaspoons or medicine spoons – to put tablets into a patient's mouth without contaminating the medication
- tissues – to cut up tablets in if necessary
- pestle and mortar – to crush tablets if necessary (NB: check with pharmacist that a liquid form is not available, and that the tablet is suitable to be crushed)

● tablet file or cutter or knife – to divide a tablet evenly (NB: check with pharmacist that smaller doses are not available and that the tablet is suitable for cutting)

● note pad – to keep a record of actions that are to be taken as a result of medication, e.g. re-ordering medication or discharge drugs, or returning to check BP or peak expiratory flow

● drug reference book, e.g. BNF – to check unfamiliar doses or drugs.

Intervention: oral drug administration

1. Wash and dry hands.
2. Consult Mr Jenkins' prescription sheet. For regular drug administration times, work systematically from the front page of the prescription sheet to identify the following issues:
   – Has Mr Jenkins any known allergies?
   – What medication is due, e.g. regular doses? When was it last given?
   – Once-only prescriptions, such as pre-medications: when are they due, or have they been given?
   – Variable doses – these may need to be updated as a result of blood tests; therefore, are they current? Check date.
   – Is analgesia required? If so, when was the last dose and was it effective? If opioids are prescribed, has the patient had all the doses, or should the analgesia needs be reviewed?
   – Progress of any current intravenous therapy – if a patient has an intravenous infusion in place, then it is an ideal opportunity to check (a) that it is running to time and (b) sufficient is prescribed for the patient's needs over the next shift (see Chapter 7).
3. Check each medication prescribed for dose, time, date, route and doctor's signature.
4. Select the medicine bottle, checking the name of the drug with that on the prescription sheet. If Mr Jenkins needs to have a pre-medication check of pulse, blood pressure or peak expiratory flow, now is the time to do that.
5. Calculate the dose.
6. Tip the required number of tablets into the lid of the container (Figure 6.1). If working with another nurse, show the name of the container and the number of tablets to the other person, stating the written dose aloud.

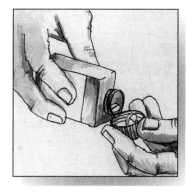

Figure 6.1
Decanting tablets
into container lid.

7. Tip the dose into the pot. If measuring liquid: ensure the lid is on firmly and then shake the bottle to ensure the contents are well mixed. Put the pot on a level surface, pour the liquid into it, turning the bottle label away so that it does not get dripped on and obscured by medicine. Pour to the required level (Figure 6.2).

TIP! **If medicine needs to be dissolved before you give it to the patient, put it into a disposable cup and let it dissolve whilst you are checking the other medicines and preparing him.**

8. Take the medication to Mr Jenkins.
9. Greet Mr Jenkins by name and check identity against the prescription sheet label.
10. Assist Mr Jenkins into an upright position to aid swallowing.
11. Ensure he understands the sequential order to take the medication; for example, antacids are taken after other tablets. Provide a

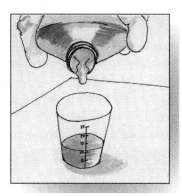

Figure 6.2
Measuring liquid
dose.

drink, and assist him to take the medication, offering tablets on a spoon if required. Ensure all medicines are taken before you leave Mr Jenkins. Do not leave any medicines beside the bed to be taken later. They may get forgotten, knocked over, or consumed accidentally by someone else.

12. Document the drug dose and time. If Mr Jenkins has refused the medication or is nil by mouth, record on the prescription sheet the reasons for withholding the dose according to the local policy code. Report to medical staff.

13. Dispose of waste and used containers.

14. Monitor Mr Jenkins for effects such as degree of pain relief, or side effects such as nausea or rashes, and document as necessary.

TIP! Strong-tasting liquids are more palatable if taken through a straw as they do not come into contact with so many taste buds.

If patients are reluctant to take their medication, crushing their tablets and putting them into food or drink may change the action of the drug. The UKCC (2001) advises that disguising medication in food or drink may be justified as being in the patient's best interests if the patient is refusing medication, but not if the patient is sufficiently rational to make an informed consent to treatment. It should not be done as a regular practice but only as a contingency measure, and never for the convenience of health care professionals.

Sublingual and buccal medications

These are designed to be released slowly by dissolving in the mouth and absorbed through the oral mucosa. The same procedure is followed as above, but for a sublingual medication such as glycerine trinitrate (GTN) the tablet is positioned under the tongue (Figure 6.3). Some patients may place a GTN tablet under the tongue to relieve angina, and when the pain has reduced, may then swallow the tablet to allow it to be absorbed more slowly. Not all sublingual drugs can be taken like this, and swallowing the tablet is usually contraindicated. Patients should therefore not drink until after the drug has dissolved; consequently, if sublingual drugs are to be taken, administer them after other medications.

Buccal medication is positioned between the gum and the cheek, and can be placed beside either the upper or lower jaw (Figure 6.4). The position should be changed each time to prevent local irritation

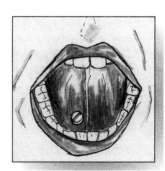

Figure 6.3
Sublingual tablet.

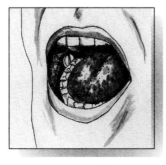

Figure 6.4
Buccal tablet.

occurring. The patient should not drink until after the tablet has dissolved. Therefore, all other medication should be taken first.

TIP! When checking sublingual or buccal tablets, put them into a separate pot from the other tablets so that they are easily identifiable and are not swallowed by mistake.

Evaluation

Did Mr Jenkins manage to take his oral medication? Do you need to find alternative preparations?

NURSING PROBLEM 6.2

Patient history: Mrs Easton has suffered a stroke and is unable to swallow (dysphagia). She cannot take anything by mouth.

Problem: Mrs Easton cannot take medication orally and requires medication via nasogastric (NG) and intramuscular (IM) routes.

Goal: Mrs Easton will safely receive medication via NG and IM routes.

Nasogastric drug administration

This route is effective for patients who cannot swallow, but whose gastrointestinal tract is functioning. It enables patients to take medication without experiencing unnecessary injections and so reduces the risks associated with intravenous therapy (see Chapter 7). Drug absorption rate is the same as the oral route, but some drugs may be less effective if not prepared correctly. Naysmith and Nicholson (1998) identify four considerations when administering nasogastric drugs:

- choice of preparation
- timing
- drug interaction with enteral feeds
- administration via the tube.

Choice of preparation

Ideally, the medication should be in liquid form. Should a liquid preparation not be available, some tablets will dissolve or the pharmacy may be able to prepare a suspension. Capsules may be aspirated by needle and syringe or dissolved in water, and the liquid administered. Granular capsules may be opened and mixed with water. Tablets may be crushed in a pestle and mortar or between two spoons. All tablet residues should be mixed with water and drawn up into a syringe for administration to ensure the correct dose is given.

ALERT!

Enteric-coated medications, modified-release preparations and some hormones and cytotoxic drugs should not be crushed as it changes the chemical actions of the drugs. It is imperative to check with the pharmacist the preferred way of preparing each of these types of medication to ensure that the drug is given correctly.

Timing

If medication should be taken on an empty stomach, it is advisable to stop the feed for 30 minutes before administration, and resume the feed 30 minutes afterwards. The exception to this is Phenytoin (Naysmith and Nicholson 1998), which requires a break from feeding for two hours before and after the feed to allow full absorption of the drug.

Interaction with the feed

Drugs should not be added directly to the feed and given simultaneously as a chemical reaction with the feed may occur, blocking the tube. To avoid potential infection from entering the feed, medication and feed should not be mixed together.

Administration procedure

Equipment

- Water container (sterile water may be the preferred requirement in some acute Trusts).
- 50 ml bladder syringe or luer lock syringe depending on type of NG tube.
- 20 ml luer lock syringe and needles.
- pH indicator paper.
- Receiver.
- Medication pot with prescribed medications.
- Container for mixing medication.
- Clamp for NG tube.
- Cap for NG administration tube.
- Absorbent pad or towel.

Procedure

The procedure described above for oral medication (page 102) for administering a drug should be followed, but with the following additional considerations:

1. Wash your hands and take the prescribed medication to Mrs Easton. Check her identity.
2. Position Mrs Easton in a semi-recumbent position to reduce reflux. Explain the procedure to her and provide privacy. Protect the pillow with a towel or absorbent pad to catch any drips.
3. Turn off the feed and clamp the NG tube. Cap the administration tube and put to one side, ensuring that the tube does not get contaminated from other surfaces.

4. Confirm the position of the NG tube in the stomach by aspirating gastric contents and checking pH (see Chapter 9). Clamp the NG tube.

5. Prepare the medication. After crushing the tablets, mix them with 15–20 ml of water and draw up into the smaller syringe, rinsing the pestle with water to ensure a full dose.

TIP! If using liquid preparations, pour them into the measuring cup one at a time. Do not mix medications in the same container: if some is spilt, you will have no way of determining what drugs have or have not been given.

6. Attach the bladder syringe or the larger luer lock syringe without the piston attachment to the NG tube. This will act as a funnel. Hold the syringe slightly above Mrs Easton's nose height to prevent backflow.

TIP! NG tubes can be clamped by kinking the tubing to prevent air from entering the patient's stomach (Figure 6.5).

7. Slowly pour the medication from the small syringe or cup into the barrel of the larger syringe, ensuring that the large syringe is held upright, and unclamp the NG tube. Raise the tube to speed the flow (Figure 6.6.1) or lower the height of the syringe to slow the flow (Figure 6.6.2). To prevent air from entering the patient's stomach, add fluid to the larger syringe before it empties completely. If resistance is felt or the tube is blocked, do not force the flow. Check the position of the NG tube by aspiration, and

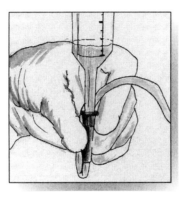

Figure 6.5
Kinking
nasogastric tube.

flushing with additional water in case a drug particle has obstructed the NG tube.

8. Flush with 5–10 ml of water between each drug, and 30–50 ml on completion of administration, now allowing the tube to empty.
9. Clamp the tube and remove syringe.
10. Reconnect to the feeding pump if required, ensuring the cap is removed from the administration set.
11. Position Mrs Easton comfortably before leaving her.
12. Document the drugs given and record the amount of fluid given on the fluid balance chart.
13. Wash equipment and dispose of all waste.

Controlled drugs

These are drugs whose prescription and use is governed by the Misuse of Drugs Act (1971), as they are potentially addictive. In the hospital setting, controlled drugs (CDs) are ordered by a registered nurse, in a duplicated order book, which must be signed when receiving drugs

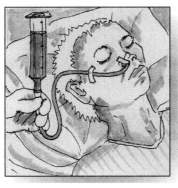

Figure 6.6.1

Figure 6.6.2

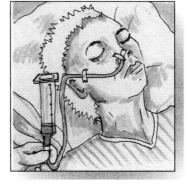

Figure 6.6.1–2 Raising and lowering NG tube.

from pharmacy. Each administration of CDs is recorded in a record book kept solely for that purpose. Both the order book and record book must be retained for two years after completion.

Security of controlled drugs

Controlled drugs are stored in the clinical area in a designated secure locked cupboard, which is used only for CDs and to which access is restricted. The nurse in charge of the area usually holds the keys but may delegate responsibility for them, therefore delegating the security of all medications to another nurse during the shift. It is essential that these keys are kept on a specific person at all times and never left lying around, for example, in a drawer or on a worktop. Routine checks of the CD stock may be made at regular intervals in a clinical area, depending on local policy, to ensure that the stock tallies with the record book. Each page should be a record of only one drug.

To check and administer a controlled drug

- Two people should be involved in the administration procedure of all controlled drugs, and where these two are nurses, one must be a registered nurse.
- The prescription is checked as for usual medication. In addition, consider the time of the previous dose of controlled drug – is it within the prescribed time period? Has the patient already received his allotted dose?
- Take the appropriate drug from the locked cupboard and compare it with the prescription sheet. Verify the dose and name of the drug. Check the quantity in the box with the record book and remove the drug from the container. Check that the remaining ampoules or tablets tally with the record book, and return the remainder to the cupboard and lock it.
- Check the dose required, route, time, and patient's identity on the prescription.
- Prepare the appropriate amount of drug required, discarding any excess in the sink.
- In the controlled drug record book, document (a) the patient details, (b) date and time, (c) dose given, (d) dose discarded, and (e) the amount of remaining stock.

- Both persons should go to the bedside, where the patient's identity should be confirmed and the prescription dose, time and route should be checked again.
- Administer the medication by the prescribed route, and document this on the prescription sheet and in the controlled drug record.

There should be no cancellation of entries, but if corrected they should be countersigned and cross-referenced if incorrect. Entries should be indelible, and the book should not be used for any other purpose.

Intramuscular (IM) injections

Injections deliver medication directly into the body and are not retrievable. It is essential, therefore, to be accurate in identifying safe entry points for injections, and to take the utmost care in administering medication by the parenteral route. The intramuscular route delivers injections directly into muscles which have an efficient blood supply and can absorb from 1 ml to 5 ml of medication, depending on the site.

Considerations before administration by the IM route

- The patient's age: elderly patients may have muscle wasting which may limit the choice of site, and babies who are not yet walking may have underdeveloped muscles, particularly in the buttocks.
- General physical status: emaciated or cachectic (extremely debilitated) patients may also have muscle wasting or poor perfusion and skin condition. Oedematous limbs will not absorb medication as effectively as those with good perfusion.
- The drug therapy: the amount to be given, and the frequency and consistency of medication will influence the choice of location. For example, a depot injection (long-term slow-release action) will require a deep muscle, to allow sufficient slow absorption over a period of time.

Assessment of appropriate site

There are five sites that may be used for IM injections: deltoid (Figure 6.7); dorso-gluteal (Figure 6.8); ventro-gluteal (Figure 6.9); and the thigh muscles – vastus lateralis and rector femoris (Figures 6.11.1–2).

Prior to injection, the proposed site should be inspected for signs of inflammation, swelling or infection; areas of skin damage should be avoided. If a course of injections are to be given then a record of each site should be documented to avoid using the same area too frequently, as complications such as muscle atrophy or a sterile abscess may occur (Springhouse 1993).

Locating deltoid site

The densest part of the muscle can be located on the mid-lateral aspect of the arm in line with the axilla, and about 2.5 cm below the acromial process (Figure 6.7). This avoids the radial nerve and brachial artery. Positioning the hand on the hip causes the muscle to relax and makes it easier to access (Workman 1999). The typical absorption volume is no greater than 1–2 ml.

Dorso-gluteal site

The patient should lie either on their side with knees slightly bent, or prone with toes pointing inwards (Figure 6.8). An imaginary line is drawn across from the cleft of the buttock to the greater trochanter of the femur. Then a vertical line is drawn midway across the first line, and the outer quadrant is identified. This quadrant is then divided into four quadrants: the desired location is the upper outer quadrant (Campbell 1995). The aim is to access the gluteus maximus muscle, and to avoid the sciatic nerve and gluteal artery. The typical absorption volume is 2–4 ml.

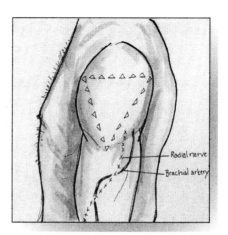

Figure 6.7
Deltoid site.

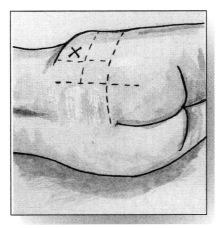

Figure 6.8
Dorso-gluteal
site.

Ventro-gluteal site

The patient can lie on either side with knees slightly flexed. Place the palm of your right hand onto the left greater trochanter (or right hand onto left hip), and extend the index finger towards the superior iliac crest. If you have small hands, start with the palm of the hand on the greater trochanter, and slide the hand up until the tip of the index finger touches the iliac crest (Covington and Trattler 1997). Stretch out middle finger to form a V and the injection should be located into the centre of the V. This will enter the gluteus medius and minimus muscles (Figure 6.9). There have been very few complications documented from the accurate use of this site (Beyea and Nicholl 1995). The typical absorption volume is 2–4 ml.

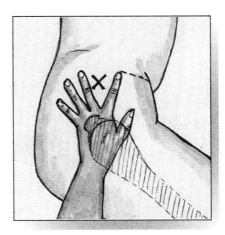

Figure 6.9
Ventro-gluteal
site.

Figure 6.10 shows the proximity of the dorso-gluteal site to the ventro-gluteal site.

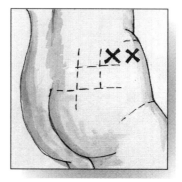

Figure 6.10
Proximity of DG and VG sites to each other.

Vastus lateralis and rector femoris

These quadriceps muscles (Figures 6.11.1–2) are particularly good for toddlers or patients who have wasted muscles as they can be 'bunched up' before injecting (Figure 6.12; Springfield 2000). They can be located by measuring a hand's breadth down from the greater trochanter, and a hand's breadth up from the knee, identifying the middle third of the muscle as the safe location. The vastus lateralis is located on the side of the leg, and the rector femoris is at the front of the thigh. The typical absorption volume is 1–4 ml.

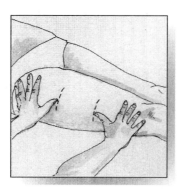

Figure 6.11.1
Vastus lateralis site.

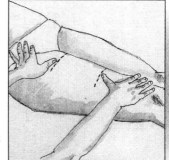

Figure 6.11.2
Rector femoris site.

Figure 6.11.1–2 Locating vastus lateralis and rector femoris sites.

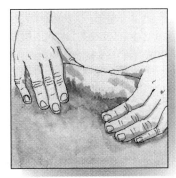

Figure 6.12
Bunched-up
muscle.

Intervention: intramuscular (IM) injection

Equipment

- 2 ml or 5 ml syringe (depending on amount for injection).
- 2 × 21 (green) or 23 (blue) gauge needle. Note: a large needle should be used for adults to ensure that it reaches the muscle layer. Short needles may result in the injection going into the adipose tissue, resulting in reduced effectiveness (Cockshott et al. 1982).
- Alcohol wipe – if required by Trust policy.
- Gauze swab.
- Receiver.
- Prescribed drug and prescription sheet.
- Gloves – to protect from drug spillage and body fluids.
- Apron – if required by Trust policy for protection as above.

Preparing the injection

This is an aseptic procedure (see Chapter 11) and therefore all equipment should be sterile. Every effort should be made to prevent contamination of equipment during the procedure.

- Check all equipment to ensure it is sealed and used within expiry date.
- Wash hands and put on gloves.
- Prepare drug vial. Carry out the same checks as described in the procedure for oral drug administration (page 102). If a glass ampoule is used, flick the top of the ampoule to encourage all fluid to drain into the reservoir. Use a tissue or piece of gauze to protect your fingers from glass cuts when breaking the top off the

ampoule. If a vial with a rubber bung is being used, remove the cover using scissors or forceps to prevent injury to your fingers; clean the rubber bung with an alcohol wipe.

● Assemble needle and syringe, taking care not to touch the needle, except for the barrel when connected to the syringe.

● Uncap the needle. It is best practice *never* to resheath an un-capped needle, even if unused, to prevent needlestick injuries.

To dilute a drug – if the drug requires mixing with a diluent, or if you are drawing fluid from a closed vial – draw up the equivalent amount of air into the syringe, steady the vial on a flat surface with one hand, and insert the syringe into the vial and inject the vial with the air (Figure 6.13). This will make it easier to withdraw. The vial can be gently rolled on the palm of the hand to aid mixing. Ensure drug is dissolved before aspirating the medication into the syringe.

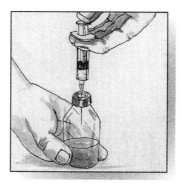

Figure 6.13
Inserting air into vial.

TIP! When drawing up a drug keep the needle bevel under the fluid level at all times to reduce the amount of air drawn up in the syringe. Adjust the angle of needle and syringe to a V shape (Figure 6.14) while drawing up.

Withdraw required amount into the syringe. Remove the vial, and holding the syringe with the needle uppermost, tap the syringe firmly to encourage air bubbles to rise to the top to be expelled. Larger syringes may have the connection on the side, rather than the middle of the syringe. To aid the air to rise to the top, tip the syringe to a slight angle so that the air collects under the connection, and keep it at that angle until all the air is expelled (Figure 6.15). This ensures an accurate dose.

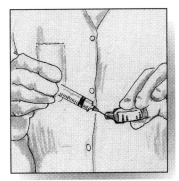

Figure 6.14
V-shape to draw
up injection.

Figure 6.15
Expelling air
from syringe.

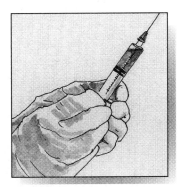

Change the needle. This ensures that the injection is given with a clean, dry, sharp needle thus reducing pain (Beyea and Nicholl 1995), and prevents a possible sharps injury resulting from transporting the injection to the patient.

TIP! Recheck the amount of dose in the syringe after you have expelled the air to make sure that you still have the right amount in the syringe and did not lose any when changing the needle. If the dose is very small do not expel the air until after you have changed the needle so that there is minimum wastage.

Administering the injection

The reason for the injection should be explained to Mrs Easton, so that she can give her verbal consent. This may be done prior to preparing the injection in case Mrs Easton would like to prepare herself, for example, by visiting the toilet or warning her visitors.

Procedure

- Take the prepared injection and prescription sheet to Mrs Easton's bedside.
- Call Mrs Easton by name, and confirm her identity and consent.
- Close the curtains to provide privacy, and assist Mrs Easton into an appropriate position depending on the chosen injection site, draping the bed and her nightclothes to protect her dignity but allowing access to the site.
- Locate the site by identifying the anatomical landmarks and encourage the patient to relax.
- If local policy dictates, the skin should be cleaned with an alcohol swab for 30 seconds and allowed to dry for 30 seconds (Simmonds 1983). If the patient is physically clean and the nurse maintains hand hygiene and asepsis during the procedure, additional skin preparation may not be necessary.
- Remove the needle cap, stretch the skin taut with thumb and index finger of your non-dominant hand.
- Position the needle just above the skin at a 90° angle, holding the syringe barrel like a dart.
- Warn Mrs Easton that she will feel a sharp prick.
- Insert the needle three-quarters of its length in, using a dart-like action.
- Aspirate to allow any blood to surface. Should any blood appear, remove the needle and discard the injection. The procedure will have to be recommenced. Continuing with the injection could result in the injection being given intravenously.
- If no blood is aspirated, proceed with the injection, injecting slowly at a rate of approximately 1 ml in 10 seconds. On completion, allow about 10 seconds before removing the needle to allow the muscle to accommodate the fluid (Beyea and Nicholl 1995).
- Remove the needle at a 90° angle and place in the receiver. Apply gentle pressure to the site with gauze.
- Make Mrs Easton comfortable. Ensure she can reach the call bell should she require any assistance, and that she has all she needs at hand. Draw the curtains.
- Remove all equipment and dispose of sharps safely. Discard apron and gloves.

- Record the dose on the prescription chart. Document additional information, such as choice of site and effect of medication in the nursing notes.

Z track technique

The Z track technique was originally used for drugs that stain the skin or are particularly irritant. Beyea and Nicholl (1995) recommend it as a method to reduce pain and leakage from intramuscular sites.

- Following location of site use the thumb to pull the skin about 3 cm to one side (Figure 6.16).
- Insert the needle at 90°, release the thumb.
- Administer the injection as above.
- Return the thumb to retract the skin, and then remove the needle.
- Remove thumb and allow skin to return to usual position.

TIP! **Twelve steps towards a painless injection (Workman 1999):**

1. **Prepare patients with appropriate information before the procedure, to aid their compliance and cooperation.**
2. **Change the needle after preparation and before administration to ensure it is clean, dry and sharp and the correct length to enter muscle layer.**
3. **Make the ventro-gluteal site the preferred choice to ensure the medication reaches the muscle layer.**
4. **Position the patient so that the chosen muscle is flexed.**

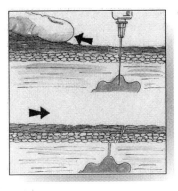

Figure 6.16
Z track
technique.

5. If cleaning the skin before injecting, ensure it is dry before injecting as alcohol can cause stinging.
6. Consider using ice or freezing spray to numb the skin before injecting, particularly for needle-phobic patients or children.
7. Use the Z track technique.
8. Rotate injection sites and document so that no one site is overused.
9. Enter the skin firmly with a controlled thrust, positioning the needle at an angle of 90° to prevent shearing and tissue displacement (Katsma and Smith 1997).
10. Inject medication steadily and slowly – about 1 ml per 10 seconds – to allow the muscle to accommodate the fluid.
11. Wait 10 seconds after completion of the injection to allow diffusion through the muscle. Then remove the needle at the same angle as it entered.
12. Apply gentle pressure but to prevent local tissue irritation do not massage the site afterwards.

Evaluation

Did Mrs Easton receive her medication by the most effective route?

NURSING PROBLEM 6.3

Patient history: Mrs Bell is a young woman who has just been diagnosed with Type 1 insulin-dependent diabetes mellitus.

Problem: Mrs Bell needs to learn how to administer her insulin subcutaneously.

Goal: Mrs Bell will be able to safely administer her insulin subcutaneously.

Subcutaneous (SC) injections

Small amounts of medication (0.2–2 ml) are given into the subcutaneous tissue to allow a slow, sustained absorption of medication. It is an ideal route for insulin, which requires frequent injections, but is also used regularly for heparin. Preferred sites for self-administered SC injections are the outer upper arms, the upper thighs, and the lower abdomen around the umbilicus (Figure 6.17). Nurses can also use the back of the upper arms, outer thighs and upper buttocks but these are not accessible for self-administration.

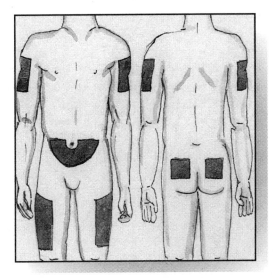

Figure 6.17
Subcutaneous injection sites.

If SC medications are administered into the muscle, it will increase the absorption rate of the drug and in the case of insulin may result in hypoglycaemia: it is important, therefore, to ensure the injection does not go too deep.

Intervention: administering subcutaneous injections

Equipment

- Insulin syringe or 1 ml syringe. If injecting insulin use an insulin syringe with a 25 or 27 gauge needle. (Patients may prefer to use an insulin pen of which there are several types.)
- 2 × 25 or 27 gauge needles (orange).
- Gauze swab.
- Receiver.
- Prescribed drug and prescription sheet.

Preparing an insulin drug dose

Preparing an insulin dose may require drawing up from more than one multi-dose vial. The following procedure explains how to do this, and allows you to draw up from an ampoule that has a vacuum in it. If the air were not injected first, it would be very difficult to withdraw insulin as the vacuum within the ampoule would draw in the contents of the syringe and cause mixing of the two different types.

To prepare an injection from two multi-dose vials (Figure 6.18):

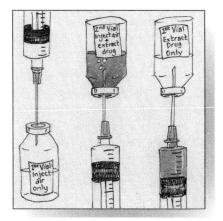

Figure 6.18
Drawing up from a multi-dose vial.

- Clean the rubber bung on both vials with an alcohol wipe.
- Draw air into the syringe to equal the volume of drug to be withdrawn from the first vial.
- With the first vial on a flat surface, insert the needle into the first vial. *Do not* touch the liquid with the needle, but inject the air and remove the needle.
- Draw air into the syringe to equal the volume of drug to be withdrawn from the second vial, insert into the second vial, and inject the air. Then invert the vial and withdraw the required dose, tap to remove air bubbles and expel, and remove needle from vial.
- Return to first vial, clean rubber bung, insert needle, invert vial and withdraw required amount carefully. Remove needle and expel air, taking care not to lose any of the first drug.
- If necessary change the needle before administration. Some disposable insulin syringes have an integral needle which cannot be changed. This is the only time that you would resheath the needle

to prevent (a) needlestick injury during transportation to the patient, and (b) contamination of sterile equipment (Figure 6.19).

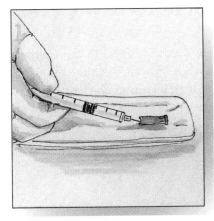

Figure 6.19
One-handed resheathing of needle.

Procedure

The first stages of the procedure are the same as those described for oral drug administration (page 102).

- Take equipment to Mrs Bell and confirm her identity. Provide privacy.
- Locate site. Do not use if there is swelling, redness, bruising or lumps. Patients that use insulin should be taught to systematically rotate within an anatomical area, as absorption rate varies depending on anatomical location (Peragallo-Dittko 1997). Other medications given subcutaneously such as heparin should also be rotated within an area to reduce bruising.
- Pinch up a fold of skin to lift the adipose tissue away from the muscle, and insert insulin needle at 90°.

WARNING!

If not using insulin equipment for SC injection the needle is longer and therefore needle entry should be at 45°.

- Release the skin fold and inject slowly and steadily.

- Withdraw needle, and if bleeding occurs apply light pressure with gauze swab.
- Discard equipment.
- Document which site has been used and record administration of the drug.

TIP! **SC injections do not require skin cleansing beforehand, provided the patient is physically clean. Also, you don't need to aspirate before injecting as the risk of puncturing a blood vessel is remote (Peragallo-Dittko 1997).**

Evaluation

Mrs Bell is able to administer subcutaneous insulin correctly.

NURSING PROBLEM 6.4

Problem: Mr Elland requires rectal medication to treat an inflamed colon.

Goal: Mr Elland will safely receive rectal medication to relieve discomfort.

Rectal medication

Rectal medication bypasses the upper gastro-intestinal tract, avoiding liver metabolism and therefore working quickly. It is suitable for patients who are unconscious, unable to swallow or are vomiting. Drugs given by suppository or enema can produce a local effect – e.g. to relieve constipation or treat local inflammation – or can work systemically – e.g. to provide pain relief.

Before administering medications rectally you should check the anal area to ensure there are no signs of rectal bleeding, skin tags, recent anorectal surgery, undiagnosed abdominal pain or paralytic ileus (Addison et al. 2000), as the procedure may aggravate these conditions. An unhurried and gentle approach should be taken to administering medication rectally, because the procedure can induce vagal stimulation resulting in bradycardia and vasodilation (Campbell 1994), and on rare occasions may cause the patient to collapse.

Intervention: administering suppositories

Equipment

- Tray.
- Prescribed suppositories – as per prescription or by group protocol.
- Disposable gloves and apron.
- Lubricant: either water for glycerine suppositories, or water-based lubricant.
- Tissues or gauze swabs.
- Protective bed cover such as incontinence pad.
- Waste disposal bag.
- Easy access to toilet, bedpan or commode.

Procedure

- Prepare to administer medications as described for oral administration of drugs (page 102).
- Wash hands and prepare equipment.
- Prepare Mr Elland. Ask Mr Elland to empty his bladder to reduce pelvic discomfort. If the medication is for systemic effect, ask him to empty his bowel if he is able. This will ensure an empty rectum and facilitate absorption. He should give his verbal consent to treatment. Encourage Mr Elland to relax as much as possible by providing privacy and ensuring that interruptions are prevented.
- Position Mr Elland on his left side, so allowing the direction of the suppository to follow the natural direction of the GI tract. Bend his knees slightly to aid comfort and ease access to the anus. Cover him with a blanket to maintain dignity and warmth.
- Protect the bed by placing the incontinence pad under his buttocks. This will reduce Mr Elland's embarrassment if there is any discharge or leakage.
- Put on gloves.
- Open suppositories and place on gauze or tissue. Lubricate as advised on pack. Glycerine suppositories may be lubricated with water.
- With your left hand, lift the upper buttock and observe the anal area for evidence of local tissue damage. Encourage deep slow

breaths during the procedure should Mr Elland begin to feel uncomfortable, and warn him that he will feel the suppository inserted.

● Insert suppository. If it is to treat constipation it should be inserted with the pointed end first (Figure 6.20.1), pushing the suppository in with the index finger along the rectal wall until it passes the internal sphincter (Springhouse 2000). It should rest next to the rectal mucosa and not in faecal matter or it will be ineffective (Campbell 1994). If the medication is for systemic effect, inserting it blunt end first (Figure 6.20.2) will reduce the patient's urge to defaecate, and aid absorption (Addison et al. 2000). If more than one suppository is ordered, repeat procedure.

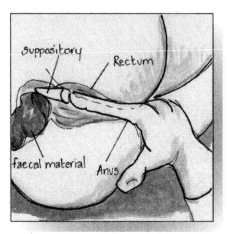

Figure 6.20.1
Constipation is treated by inserting suppositories pointed end first.

Figure 6.20.2
Blunt end of suppository inserted first for systemic effect

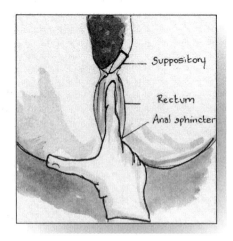

Figure 6.20.1–2 Insertion of suppository.

- Gentle pressure on the anal area with a gauze or tissue pad will reduce the desire for immediate defaecation. Encourage Mr Elland to retain the suppository for as long as possible (at least 20 minutes) for it to be effective, and to rest on his side for at least five minutes to aid retention.
- Clean perineal area with tissues.
- Dispose of all waste, removing gloves by turning inside out to prevent cross-contamination.
- Wash hands.
- Record administration on the prescription sheet and document the outcome.

 TIP! **Suppositories are easier to administer if kept in the fridge until required unless otherwise stated on the drug information sheet.**

Intervention: administering enemas

Equipment

- Disposable gloves and apron.
- Prescribed enema and prescription sheet.
- Lubrication.
- Bowl/receiver of warm water.
- Gauze swabs or tissues.
- Waste bag.
- Protective bed cover or incontinence pad.
- Easy access to toilet, bedpan or commode.

Procedure

- Prepare to administer medications as described for oral administration of drugs (page 102).
- Wash hands and prepare equipment.
- At the bedside remove outer packaging from the enema if necessary and place in warm water to raise it to room temperature to reduce shock and bowel spasms. Retention enemas are usually 200 ml or less to promote retention (Addison et al. 2000).
- Prepare Mr Elland. Ask Mr Elland to empty his bladder to reduce pelvic discomfort. If the medication is for systemic effect, ask him to empty his bowel if he is able, to ensure an empty rectum and

facilitate absorption (Heywood Jones 1995). He should give his verbal consent to treatment. Encourage Mr Elland to relax as much as possible by providing privacy and ensuring interruptions are prevented.

- Position him on his left side, so allowing the enema to flow in the natural direction of the GI tract. Bend his knees slightly to aid comfort and ease access to the anus. Cover him with a blanket to maintain dignity and warmth.
- If administering a steroid enema, the patient's bed should have the bottom raised to a 45° angle to help retention. Patients receiving steroid retention enemas are likely to have them administered at bedtime to enable the medication to be absorbed overnight whilst resting (Addison et al. 2000).
- Protect the bed by placing the incontinence pad under his buttocks. This will reduce Mr Elland's embarrassment if there is any discharge or leakage.
- Put on gloves.
- Ensure enemas are mixed by gentle shaking before administration.
- Place lubricant on clean gauze and apply to the enema tube. Using fluid from the enema to lubricate the tube may cause local irritation to the anus.
- Remove the plastic tip from the nozzle of the enema.
- Expel air through the tube by rolling up the enema bag from the base.
- Warn Mr Elland that you are about to give the enema and that he will feel the tube and gentle pressure in the rectum. Suggest that he takes deep breaths and tries to relax during the procedure.
- Lift the upper buttock and gently insert the enema tube into the anus as far along the tube as possible, and allow the fluid to flow into the rectum by gravity (Addison et al. 2000). Roll up the bag as the fluid flows in, to prevent backflow. Tube extensions are available for self-administration (Heywood Jones 1995).
- Gentle pressure on the anal area with a gauze or tissue pad will reduce the desire for immediate defaecation. Encourage Mr Elland to retain the enema for as long as possible (5–15 minutes for evacuant enemas) for it to be effective, and to rest on his side for at least five minutes to aid retention. Retention medicated enemas should be retained for at least 30–60 minutes or as long as the patient can hold onto them (Springhouse 2000).

- Clean perineal area with tissues.
- Ensure easy access to toileting facilities.
- Dispose of all waste, removing gloves by turning inside out to prevent cross-contamination.
- Wash hands.
- Record administration on the prescription sheet and document the outcome. Record any additional observations such as the consistency, appearance and quantity of stools.

TIP! **Caution should be taken with administering phosphate enemas to elderly or debilitated patients as complications such as trauma to local tissue can occur, causing bleeding. There may be local irritation, or on rare occasions a systemic reaction (Addison et al. 2000).**

Evaluation

Did Mr Elland receive his suppository or enema without discomfort? What was the effect of the medication?

NURSING PROBLEM 6.5

Patient history: Mrs Paur is an elderly lady with many medical problems, one of which is glaucoma.

Problem: Mrs Paur requires eye drops to treat glaucoma.

Goal: Mrs Paur will have her eye drops administered safely.

Ophthalmic medication

Ophthalmic medication is usually applied topically, the most common methods being eye drops or ointment. These may be used for diagnostic purposes such as dilating the pupil prior to examination; anaesthetizing the eye prior to treatment, or for treatment of eye conditions such as glaucoma or infection.

Heywood Jones (1995) recommends that administration of ophthalmic medication follows these principles:

- Always use separately labelled drug containers for each eye to prevent cross-infection.
- If eye drops and ointment are prescribed to be administered at the same time, give the drops first, then administer ointment several minutes later, as the ointment can prevent absorption of the drops.
- Medication should not be directed onto the cornea of the eye as this may damage the cornea, but directed into the area in the lower eyelid (Figure 6.21).

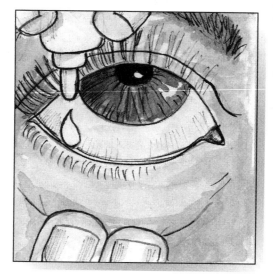

Figure 6.21
Eye drops directed into lower eyelid.

- When clearing discharge from the eye or wiping away excess medication, do not use dry cotton-wool balls as fibres may get into the eye and damage the cornea.
- Always work from the inner canthus (nose side) outwards to edge of eye when applying ointment or swabbing eye to reduce infection risk.
- Medication containers should not touch the eye during administration as they may become contaminated or damage the eye.
- Once an eye medication has been opened, record the starting date on the container and discard after two weeks.
- If both eyes are to be treated but only one is discharging, treat the cleaner eye first to prevent cross-infection. Wash hands between eyes.

TIP! A patient who is receiving eye medication may have some visual impairment. Always introduce yourself to him as you approach, so that you can be identified by your voice even if his sight is limited.

Intervention: administering eye medication

Equipment

- Prescribed medication and prescription.
- Tissues or gauze swabs.
- Sterile saline solution and sterile eye dressing pack containing gallipot and sterile gauze (if eye requires cleansing prior to drug administration).

Procedure

- Following the standard procedure for drug administration (page 102), check the prescribed medication and identify Mrs Paur, explaining the procedure and gaining her consent. Sometimes patients require different medications in each eye, so ensure you clearly identify the correct eye to receive each medication.
- Prepare equipment.
- Wash hands.
- Prepare Mrs Paur. She may prefer sitting upright in the chair, or lying on the bed with her head supported comfortably. Confirm which eye is to be treated. Give her a tissue to use after the procedure to soak up any moisture.
- If discharge is present, wash your hands, and then clean the eye using a sterile eye care pack. Swab the discharge with sterile swabs moistened with sterile saline, working from the inner canthus to the outer edge, cleaning first the upper lid, then the lower lid. Use a single swab once for each wipe to reduce potential cross-infection. Dry the eye with a gauze swab.
- Position yourself behind Mrs Paur, or to one side, so that you can place your dominant hand on her forehead, holding the medication downwards ready for application; place your other hand below the eye to pull the lower lid down gently with your index finger (Figure 6.22).

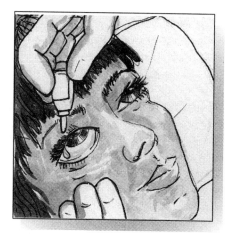

Figure 6.22
Hand positions to administer eye drops.

- Tell Mrs Paur to look upwards, so that the cornea is raised away from the site of medication delivery.
- Deliver the required number of drops into the lower lid area – nearer the outer edge to reduce drainage from the nasal tear duct. If more than one type of drug is to be administered, allow several minutes to elapse between different medications.
- If administering ointment, squeeze a length of ointment along the lower lid from the inner canthus to the outer, squeezing out additional ointment as required. To break the flow of ointment, twist the tube upwards, and stop pressing the tube. Be careful not to touch any part of the eye or eyelid as it will cause Mrs Paur to blink and interrupt the application flow.
- Remove hands and allow Mrs Paur to blink gently two or three times to disperse the medication, but do not let her squeeze her eyes.
- Dry excess moisture with tissue or sterile gauze.
- Leave Mrs Paur in a comfortable position. Advise her that her vision may be briefly impaired while her eyes respond to the medication.
- Wash hands and dispose of all waste.
- Document on the prescription sheet. Record in the nursing notes any observations regarding the state of the treated eye, such as redness, inflammation or amount of discharge.

Evaluation

Were Mrs Paur's eye drops given effectively?

Further reading

Beyea SC, Nicholl LH (1995) Administration of medications via the intramuscular route: an integrative review of the literature and research-based protocol for the procedure. Applied Nursing Research 5(1): 23–33.

British National Formulary. London: British Medical Association and British Pharmaceutical Society.

Covington TP, Trattler MR (1997) Learn how to zero in on the safest site for an IM injection. Nursing (January): 62–63.

Naysmith MR, Nicholson J (1998) Nasogastric drug administration. Professional Nurse 13(7): 424–27.

Rodger MA, King L (2000) Drawing up and administering intramuscular injections: a review of the literature. Journal of Advanced Nursing 31(3): 574–82.

Workman BA (1999) Safe injection techniques. Nursing Standard 13(39): 47–53.

UKCC (2000) Guidelines for the Administration of Medications. London: UKCC.

CHAPTER 7

Maintaining fluid balance

Barbara Workman

Aims and learning outcomes

This chapter considers the intake of fluids by the oral and parenteral routes, and details practices to be followed to ensure safe administration of fluids and blood by the intravenous route. By the end of the chapter you will be able to:

- assist a patient to increase their oral fluid intake
- accurately complete a fluid intake and output chart
- discuss factors that affect fluid balance
- identify common intravenous fluids and their uses
- prepare equipment for an intravenous infusion, monitor its progress and discontinue when appropriate
- recognize complications of IV therapy and take appropriate actions to prevent or relieve complications
- discuss the precautions that are used during a blood transfusion to ensure a safe transfusion.

Monitoring fluid balance

This is an essential aspect of nursing care because it can make a great deal of difference to the patient's comfort and recovery but requires few highly technical nursing skills. To be effective it should be accurate, otherwise assessment of the patient's condition is based on false information and may result in a patient's condition deteriorating unnecessarily (Morrison 2000).

Homeostasis is the term used to describe the balance that the body maintains between fluid intake and fluid output. It is estimated that a healthy person requires at least 2–2.5 litres, intake of fluid daily (Edwards 2001) which, together with food and metabolic processes, results in an intake of approximately 3 litres of fluid daily. Patients will vary as to how much and how often they like to drink, and some will need more encouragement than others to maintain or increase a satisfactory fluid intake. Fluid intake can be by oral drinks, food, tube feeds and intravenous fluids. Fluid output may occur via urine, vomiting, faeces and diarrhoea, sweat, gastric secretions, or wound drainage.

The lack of adequate fluid intake can lead to dehydration which presents (Morrison 2000) as:

- dry mouth and lips
- dry skin with loss of elasticity (turgor)
- weakness and lethargy
- thirst
- sunken eyes
- small concentrated urine output (oliguria)
- confusion
- tachycardia
- poor peripheral perfusion leading to pallor.

Accurate measurement of a patient's fluid intake and output will identify those patients at risk of becoming dehydrated or overhydrated. Particularly vulnerable patients are:

- the elderly, who may have lost their thirst stimulus and neglect to drink
- the confused or neurologically disordered, who may fail to respond to thirst
- those whose conditions are deteriorating, e.g. with renal or cardiac failure
- post-operative patients

- emergency admissions as their fluid needs may be initially under-estimated
- those who are nil by mouth.

Patients' fluid requirements will increase:

- in hot weather
- with a pyrexia (high temperature)
- if a urinary catheter is in situ
- if constipated
- if there is fluid loss from the gastro-intestinal tract, such as diar-rhoea, vomiting, or nasogastric or wound drainage.

Patient history

Mrs May is a 79-year-old lady who has been admitted following a fall at home. Her daughter normally drops in to see her most days, but had been away for the weekend, and found Mrs May on the floor when she came home. Her daughter says that Mrs May is very independent but has become increasingly forgetful recently, and would sometimes forget when she last had a meal. Mrs May has facial bruising and a possible head injury so has been admitted for observation.

NURSING PROBLEM 7.1

Problem: Mrs May is dehydrated.

Goal: Mrs May is to be rehydrated and to maintain an oral fluid intake of at least 2 litres per day.

Intervention: increase oral fluid intake

- Commence Mrs May on an accurate fluid balance chart. Ensure she understands that all fluid intake and output are to be measured and recorded.
- Plan to give her a drink of at least 100 ml (approximately half a glass or cup of fluid) per waking hour in addition to regular drinks provided at mealtimes, over 24 hours.

TIP! Specifying a specific amount to be consumed in a period of time will make it easier to monitor and spread the intake over the 24-hour period, and so be achievable. The equivalent of 1.5 litres is about 8 cups or 5 mugs of fluid a day (Morrison 2000).

● Ensure the drink is placed within the reach of Mrs May, and that she can pick up and hold it and is in a safe and comfortable position to consume it. Offer a feeding beaker if necessary. Assist drinking if the fluid is very hot and there is a danger of scalding.

● Offer a wide range of fluids to improve incentive to drink.

TIP! Patients who are reluctant to drink may enjoy:

- sucking ice cubes or frozen fruit juices
- very hot or very cold water in preference or in addition to tea or coffee
- savoury drinks such as diluted hot stock cubes (ensure the patient is not on a low-salt diet before offering this)
- carbonated water to relieve nausea
- fizzy drinks, which may be more palatable than tepid water that has been sitting beside a bed for a while. Ensure that the patient does not have a high intake of sugar through fluids as this will increase dehydration
- fluids drunk from a feeding beaker, which may be easier for patients with restricted movement
- fluids drunk through a straw, to relieve hiccoughs
- milk, poured on cereals or taken as milkshakes
- jellies, ice-cream, soups and thickened fluids to increase fluid intake. All of these may assist swallowing for patients with dysphagia (Leech and McDonnell 1999)
- proprietary fluid or food supplements, particularly if they are not consuming a full diet.

● Teach Mrs May about the importance of maintaining oral fluid intake to 1.5–2 litres per day. She may be reluctant to continue on this regime if she suffers from urinary urge or incontinence, so she needs to understand the importance of adequate fluid intake in preventing the urgency and frequency resulting from concentrated urine (Addison 1999).

- Record fluid intake on fluid balance chart by documenting each drink after it has been consumed, to accurately reflect intake.
- Ensure the fluid balance sheet is completed accurately at the end of each shift, and totalled every 24 hours.

TIP! **Record the amount of fluid contained in:**

a teacup

a glass

a mug

an ice cube

a soup bowl

a glass of fruit juice.

Use this to accurately monitor and record fluid intake. Evidence suggests that nurses are not sure about the quantities contained in these common containers (Morrison 2000).

Evaluation

Mrs May is no longer dehydrated, and is able to maintain a satisfactory fluid intake.

NURSING PROBLEM 7.2

Problem: Mrs May is dehydrated and has a reduced urine output.

Goal: Mrs May will be rehydrated within 24 hours, demonstrated by a urinary output of approximately 1 500 ml per day.

Urine output in health is approximately 1.5–2 litres per day (Edwards 2001). When measuring urine output hourly a patient is expected to excrete a minimum of 30 ml per hour (720 ml/day). Failure to excrete this amount per hour will have a significant impact on a patient's fluid and electrolyte balance and therefore monitoring of urine output is essential, particularly in serious illness.

Intervention: record fluid output

- Inform Mrs May that you are monitoring all her fluid intake and output to gain her cooperation.

- If Mrs May is able to use the toilet, ask if she is able to pass water directly into the measuring jug. She may find it more acceptable to pass water into a bedpan on the toilet, or use a bedpan or commode. Dispose of toilet tissue in clinical waste bag.
- Wear clean gloves and apron and use an individual measuring jug when measuring urine to prevent cross-infection (Ayliffe et al. 1999).
- Empty fluid contents of bedpan or commode into jug. Some fluid may be lost when the toilet tissue is discarded.
- In addition all fluid excreta should be monitored. Vomit should be poured into the jug to be measured. If measuring gastric aspirate, the nasogastric tube should be fully aspirated and the contents poured from the bladder syringe into the measuring jug. When no more fluid can be aspirated the amount may be measured. If small amounts of any fluid, particularly urine, are passed, accurate measurement in a jug will not be possible under 50 ml. A bladder syringe or calibrated urinometer should be used to ensure accurate measurement of small quantities.

TIP! Place jug on a level surface to read amount accurately.

- Record on fluid balance chart (see example below), and report any abnormalities to senior staff.

TIP! Contamination with solid faeces will give an inaccurate reading. Passing liquid faeces will inevitably increase fluid output; where possible the output may be measured, although accuracy will be difficult – recording of frequency alone may only be possible. If large amounts of faecal matter are lost but are essential to monitor, it is possible to record faecal weight in grams. This may be weighed by using special cartons or disposable waterproof pads. As 1 g = 1 ml, this will give some guide as to the fluid loss. A clean pad or carton should be weighed, the faeces should be poured into it from the bedpan or commode, and the pad or carton should then be weighed again. The difference in weight will equal the amount of fluid lost. Scales designated for this purpose only should be used to limit cross-infection.

Evaluation

Mrs May's urine output has returned to and is maintained at 1.5 litres a day.

Example of a fluid balance chart

This chart shows the patient is in a positive balance of 1 620 ml. The oral intake is low but the intravenous fluid compensates for this. As can be seen, the amount of intravenous fluid is being reduced towards the end of the day and then discontinued at midnight. Oral fluids should be encouraged hourly when the patient is awake to compensate for the reduction in IV fluids.

	Patient name A.N. Other . . . . Hospital Number H54321P						
	INTAKE		OUTPUT				
Time (hours)	Oral	IV	Urine	Vomit	Drainage	Other	Balance
01.00		1 litre D/Saline start					
02.00							
03.00							
04.00			350				
05.00							
06.00							
07.00							
08.00	tea 100 juice 60	D/Saline 1 000 ml given. 5% Dext 1 litre start	200				+1160 −550 = +610
09.00							
10.00	coffee 60 ml		250		25 drain removed		
11.00							

	Patient name A.N. Other . . . . Hospital Number H54321P						
	INTAKE		OUTPUT				
Time (hours)	Oral	IV	Urine	Vomit	Drainage	Other	Balance
12.00	soup 100						
13.00							
14.00							
15.00							
16.00	tea 200	5% Dext finish 1 000 ml given. 500 ml 0.9% Saline start	250				+2 520 −1 075 = +1 445
17.00							
18.00	tea 100		300				
19.00							
20.00							
21.00							
22.00	water 100						
23.00			225				
24.00	water 100	0.9% Saline 400 ml given. IVI discontinued					+3 220 −1 600 = +1 620
Total	820	2 400	1 575	Nil	25	Nil	
Balance	+3 220		−1 600				+1 620

Fluid overload

It is possible to overhydrate a patient, particularly when administering intravenous fluids. The patient may present with the following symptoms (Perry and Potter 1997; Edwards 2000):

- feeble, weak, irregular pulse
- breathlessness and cough, expectorating white or pink frothy sputum
- discomfort and restlessness
- oedema, particularly around ankles and sacrum
- lethargy
- anxiety
- distended neck veins
- raised blood pressure
- raised fluid intake and insufficient output on fluid balance chart.

Careful monitoring of a patient's fluid intake should detect these signs and symptoms early so that the fluid intake can be reduced and the fluid overload reversed. Report your observations to senior staff and medical practitioner immediately.

Peripheral intravenous therapy

Intravenous therapy (IVT) is a very common clinical intervention in modern acute care, and at least 50 per cent of patients admitted in the UK may have intravenous interventions during their stay (Wilkinson 1996). Patients receiving IVT are either unable to take fluids and medications orally to meet their needs, or these substances are not suitable to be given by the oral route. IVT by the peripheral route is an invasive procedure and all IVT care should follow aseptic principles to prevent infection. The patient's comfort and safety are of central importance during the infusion.

Spencer (1996) identifies some uses of IVT as:

- fluid and electrolyte replacement
- blood transfusion therapy
- drug administration
- parenteral nutrition.

Fluids commonly used in intravenous therapy include the following.

0.9% sodium chloride in water

This is isotonic and therefore does not encourage fluid to move from the intracellular compartments (cells) to the extracellular compartments (plasma and interstitial fluid), but replaces fluid lost from the circulation such as that lost by haemorrhage or dehydration.

Sodium chloride can be infused in other strengths to correct electrolyte imbalance, e.g. 1.8% or 3%. These concentrations are hypertonic and so draw fluid from the cells into the plasma and interstitial fluid compartments, thus increasing the fluid in circulation.

Hypotonic sodium chloride 0.45%

This can be used to correct severe dehydration arising from conditions such as diabetic ketoacidosis, and returns fluid to the cells. Too much sodium chloride by infusion can result in fluid and sodium overload, and potassium imbalance (Hand 2001), and therefore should be monitored closely.

5% dextrose in water

This isotonic fluid provides fluid replacement without disturbing the electrolyte balance and provides energy up to 170 calories in 1 litre (Hand 2001). Stronger concentrations of dextrose such as 10% or 20% may be used to provide calorie intake for patients who are temporarily unable to eat. Dextrose infusions, especially when containing potassium, are acidic and may irritate a patient's veins causing phlebitis after several days, use.

Other substances may be used to expand intravascular volume, such as:

- blood and its derivatives (see 'Blood transfusion', page 168)
- artificial colloids such as dextrans, hydroxyethyl starch (HES) and gelatin derivatives. These are used to expand the plasma volume when there have been large blood losses.

NURSING PROBLEM 7.3

Patient history: Mr Elliot is a 53-year-old man, who has been admitted with abdominal pain. He is not to have any oral food or fluids (nil by mouth) while the cause of his pain is investigated.

Problem: Mr Elliot is nil by mouth so requires fluids by intravenous infusion.

Goal: Mr Elliot will have a peripheral cannula sited and intravenous infusion administered safely.

Intervention: commencing intravenous therapy

Equipment

- Cannula – green (21G) or pink (23G) are the commonest sizes. Use the smallest size as possible, depending on the patient's treatment needs, to reduce trauma to the vein (RCN 1999).
- Antiseptic skin preparation, e.g. 2% chlorhexidine solution or 70% alcohol wipes (Ayliffe et al. 1999).
- Sterile tape and sterile dressing or designated IV dressing.
- Sterile gloves (correct size for the trained nurse or doctor inserting the cannula).
- Towel or disposable waterproof pad to protect the bed.
- Tourniquet.
- Intravenous infusion administration set.
- IV fluid as prescribed.
- Prescription sheet.
- 10 ml 0.9% saline solution to flush cannula; needle and 10 ml syringe to administer.
- Disinfectant hand rub.
- IV pole – this may be portable with casters, or fixed to the bed.
- Receiver.

Procedure

- Explain the rationale for the procedure to Mr Elliot to gain his consent and cooperation. Mr Elliot may be very anxious about this treatment since he may perceive it to mean that he is seriously ill. Information gleaned from relatives or friends may increase his anxiety (Dougherty 1996) so a clear explanation of the procedure and the expected length of therapy should be given to help to reduce his worries.
- Wash hands.
- Gather equipment in a clean tray.

TIP! Some local policies advocate the use of local anaesthetic prior to insertion of IV cannula. Anaesthetic cream should be applied at least 20–90 minutes before procedure (depending on the type used) to allow for full effect; check the manufacturer's instructions regarding this. Local anaesthetic cream may be particularly useful for patients who are afraid of needles. Injecting local anaesthetic may be as painful as siting the cannula, and the resultant localized swelling may obscure the vein (Dougherty 1998).

● Take equipment to the bedside and position the patient comfortably with easy access to the non-dominant arm. This arm should be chosen in preference, so that Mr Elliot may use his dominant arm and maintain some independence during treatment.

TIP! Avoid arms which are swollen (lymphoedema), or with open wounds. Consider cultural preferences for a 'clean' and 'dirty' hand when helping to select a vein.

● Check prescribed fluid against prescription sheet and follow the five Rs for right drug administration – Right patient, Right drug (fluid), Right route, Right time, and Right dose.
● Wash hands.
● Open the outer wrapper of the prescribed fluid. Check the container for cracks, leaks or breakage in sterility; expiry date; and check that the fluid is clear – any discolouration, particles or cloudiness indicates contamination.
● Invert the bag several times gently – but do not shake – to ensure the solution is well mixed. This is particularly important if potassium or other drugs have been added to prevent layers forming (Metheny 1990).
● Open the administration set pack and close the clamp. See Figure 7.1 for different types of clamps.
● Place the bag on a flat surface and break the protective cap off the port.
● Remove the protective cap from the administration set spike. Holding the connection port firmly in one hand, insert the spike into the port with the other hand, ensuring that the connections do not touch anything (Figure 7.2).
● Hang the bag on the IV pole and squeeze the administration set chamber to half full.
● Open the roller clamp and allow the fluid to run through the administration set into a receiver until it emerges at the end (Figure 7.3). Ensure all air bubbles are removed. Clip the end of the tubing of the administration set into the roller clamp to prevent it from being contaminated.

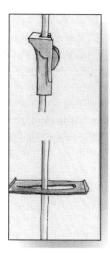

Figure 7.1 Types of IV clamp. Roller clamp.

Slide clamp.

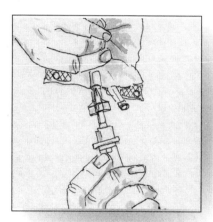

Figure 7.2 Connecting IV bag and administration set aseptically.

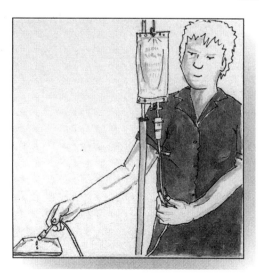

Figure 7.3 Running through administration set.

TIP! Position the roller clamp just under the chamber before attaching the administration set to the bag. This will allow you to fill the chamber and run the fluid through the administration set with the minimum of air entering the system, saving time and fluid. Air bubbles may not flush out easily and a lot of fluid may be lost as you try to remove them. Once the administration set is full, if there are air bubbles still in the tubing, give the tubing a gentle shake to dislodge the bubbles. Allow them to rise up in the tubing.

● Prepare the flush solution by drawing up the prescribed amount of 0.9% saline into a 10 ml syringe. Studies have not yet determined the optimum amount of flush solution, but experience suggests that 2–5 ml is sufficient. Place on the tray, protecting the syringe connection from contamination, and enabling the person who is cannulating to retrieve it safely and easily when ready.

● Prepare the skin for cannulation. Adequate cleansing and disinfection of the site should be undertaken by alcohol swab or using 2% aqueous chlorhexidine solution by cleansing for 30 seconds and allowing to dry for up to 1 minute (Ayliffe et al. 1999). This has been shown to be most effective at preventing cannula-related infection. If the patient is very hairy, clipping or depilatory (hair removing) cream rather than shaving is preferable as these methods do not cause skin abrasions. Following skin preparation the area should not be touched again (RCN 1999).

● To confirm patency the trained practitioner should flush the cannula with 0.9% saline solution.

● When the doctor or trained nurse has successfully cannulated the vein, remove protector from administration set and connect it to the cannula.

TIP! As connection is likely to involve contact with blood, gloves should be worn. To reduce contamination during manipulation of the IV, it is preferable for one person only to touch the area during the procedure. To reduce blood loss, press on the vein just above the cannula.

● Secure the cannula. Cannulas may be secured by sterile tape (Figure 7.4), which can be achieved by using a new roll and cutting with scissors that have been cleaned using an alcohol wipe (Workman 1999), and dressing the site with sterile gauze. (See 'Securing a cannula', page 150.) However, the usual, and increasingly preferred, method is to use a specific IV dressing which is semi-permeable to allow the site to 'breathe' and remain dry without admitting micro-organisms. It should be applied to clean dry skin, maintaining aseptic technique and not touching the sterile surface. The dressing is applied directly over the insertion site and

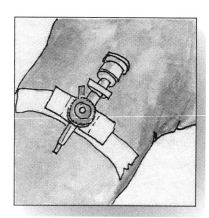

Figure 7.4.1
Place strip under cannula wings.

Figure 7.4.2
Secure each wing parallel to cannula.

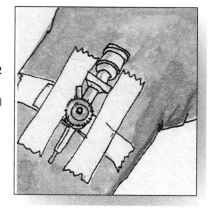

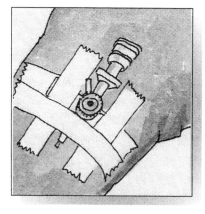

Figure 7.4.3
Tuck strip arond cannula hub.

Figure 7.4.1–3 Taping cannula.

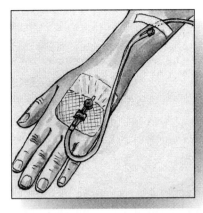

Figure 7.5
Transparent
dressing to
cannula and
securing IV set
to arm.

tucked around the hub of the cannula to ensure a firm seal, and prevent movement of the cannula (Figure 7.5).

- Secure the administration set by taping the tubing to Mr Elliot's arm (Figure 7.5) to prevent pulling on the cannula site. Bandages and/or splints should only be used in exceptional circumstances, for example, if the patient is a child or confused. If secured too tightly they can prevent the infusion from running satisfactorily, prevent regular observation of the limb, and cause stiffness and discomfort.
- Commence the infusion at the prescribed rate. Check again within the hour that the infusion is running as previously set.
- Label the administration set with the date and time of commencement, and your initials.
- Make Mr Elliot comfortable, and ensure that he has all he requires, including the call bell.
- Dispose of all equipment and wash hands.
- In the nursing notes, document: the site and size of cannula; time and date of commencement of infusion – and set rate on the fluid balance chart; and the batch number, start date, time and signatures of administering staff on the prescription sheet.

Securing a cannula

The entry site of the cannula should not come into contact with the tape as it has been found to predispose to infection. Use a clean or new roll of tape, and cut with scissors that have been cleaned, or are sterile. Using the H method, as illustrated, for cannulas with wings will secure the cannula firmly and be easy to remove, and keep the tape well away from the cannula site. This method *should only be used* if the patient is allergic to a transparent dressing, or if there are none available.

Procedure

- Cut four short strips of tape (about 5 cm long).
- Place one under the cannula wings – this protects the skin under the plastic wings (Figure 7.4.1).
- Place a strip of tape lengthways, parallel to the cannula and on each side of the cannula, securing each wing (Figure 7.4.2).
- Place the final strip of tape across the wings, tucking it around the cannula hub to secure it firmly (Figure 7.4.3).
- Apply a sterile gauze dressing over the cannula site. Write the date, time of insertion and your initials on a piece of tape and use it as a label on the dressing.
- Change the dressing daily, or more frequently if it becomes soiled or wet.

Applying a transparent semi-permeable IV dressing

The advantage of a transparent dressing is that the IV site can be observed without removing the dressing. If not applied correctly, the cannula may become loose and cause irritation to the vein. Manufacturers of sterile IV dressings do not advocate the use of tape in addition to their dressings.

- Make sure the site is clean and dry.
- Open the packaging and use aseptic technique to apply it. Peel the backing paper off the transparent end, leaving the port backing paper on.
- Position the transparent film over the entry site and apply tension to the sides of the dressing to place it smoothly in situ, tucking the film around the cannula hub to hold it firm (Figure 7.5).
- Take the rest of the backing film off and stick the wings down, allowing the film to conform to the shape of the cannula, before securing it to the skin. This will hold it firmly in place, and not pull on the skin surface.

● Change the dressing if it becomes wet underneath, soiled or loose (RCN 1999). Removing it without dislodging the cannula is very tricky. If the cannula does move while removing the dressing it will need to be resited. Do *not* try to push the cannula back into the vein as it may snap causing an embolus, may introduce infection, or may pierce the vein.

Management of an IV infusion

Intervention: regulation of flow rate

The flow rate of an infusion is determined by the amount of fluid to be given over a prescribed time. Fluid rate can be controlled manually by using a slide or roller clamp, which can be adjusted to deliver fluid at a number of drops per minute by a gravity administration set. This method will deliver approximate amounts, and therefore will not be suitable for all IV fluids. Fluids that require an exact delivery rate should be given by a syringe driver, electronic pump or mechanical pump. It is important to deliver fluids as prescribed to prevent fluid overload, and to ensure accurate drug doses.

To accurately deliver fluids the correct administration set should be selected. Check the label on the packaging to determine how many drops per minute it will deliver and the compatible type of electronic infusion device:

● standard administration set = 20 drops per ml for aqueous solutions: this set may be used with or without a compatible electronic device
● blood administration set = 15 drops per ml: this has an integral filter system but particular treatments may require additional filtration
● paediatric administration set (burette) = 60 drops per ml: a burette may also be used for adults when delivering some intravenous drugs or small amounts of fluid.

TIP! To help you understand the flow rate, when setting an IV rate, try to visualize the drops going into a teaspoon. For example, a teaspoon holds 5 ml, so an administration set giving 20 drops a ml would produce a very small amount.

Calculating flow rates

The formula for calculating IV infusion rates is as follows:

$$\frac{\text{amount of fluid}}{\text{number of hours}} \times \frac{\text{drops per ml}}{60 \text{ (minutes)}} = \text{drops per minute}$$

If calculated as in the following stages this formula uses simple figures and can be used without relying on a calculator.

1. To find out the number of ml per hour.
   Divide the total amount of fluid by the number of hours:

e.g. $\dfrac{1000 \text{ ml}}{8 \text{ hours}} = 125 \text{ ml/hour}$

TIP! This is useful to know straight away because if you are using an electronic device it usually needs to have the amount of fluid per hour set. If an electronic device is not being used, knowing how much fluid per hour is to be delivered means that you can observe the amount on the calibrations of the IV bag to monitor the accuracy of flow.

2. To calculate the number of drops per minute (dpm).
   A standard administration set gives 20 dpm, therefore divide 60 minutes by 20:

   $60 \div 20 = 3$

   A blood administration set gives 15 dpm; therefore 60 minutes ÷ 15 dpm = 4.

   A burette set gives 60 minutes ÷ 60 dpm = 1.

3. Divide the ml per hour by dpm:
   125 ml ÷ 3 = 41.6 = 42 dpm

   If using the blood administration set:
   125 ml ÷ 4 = 31 dpm

If using a burette set:

125 ml ÷ 1 = 125 dpm

When calculating the rate per hour the number should be rounded down to the nearest whole number if the answer is below 0.5 dpm, or rounded up to the next whole number if the amount is greater than 0.5 dpm.

Examples to try

Calculate the infusion rates for the following:

1. 500 ml 5% dextrose infusion in 4 hours. What should be the rate in ml per hour and drops per minute?

2. 420 ml blood. How many ml per hour and drops per minute?

TIP! **If you are uncertain about calculating flow rates, check your answers with a calculator. If you know another way to calcu-late the flow rates make sure that the answers are consis-tent, and that you can explain it to another nurse to make sure you are administering doses safely.**

Intervention: setting the flow rate manually

Equipment

- Watch with second hand.
- Prescription sheet to calculate required rate.
- IV administration set and IV fluid.

Procedure

- Calculate required rate.
- Hold the watch with the second hand next to the IV administration chamber (Figure 7.6). Use your other hand to adjust the flow by opening or closing the roller clamp.
- Set the clamp to allow fluid to flow at an approximate rate and count the drops over 15 seconds. Multiply by 4 to get an idea how

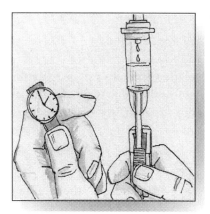

Figure 7.6
Setting flow rate.

fast the infusion is running per minute (4 × 15 = 60 seconds). Adjust the rate of flow faster or slower as required, checking the rate by the watch.

●   Before leaving the patient, confirm that the infusion is running as you have set it. Ensure the patient understands that the flow rate should only be adjusted by medical or nursing staff and that speeding it up will not result in early discontinuation of IVT (Wilkinson 1996).

●   Check flow rates: after the first hour of commencing an infusion; when administering a patient's drugs (by any route); and when undertaking any care that has involved moving the patient's position, such as turning him or providing toilet facilities. Movement may cause the cannula to change position and affect the rate of flow.

Intervention: delivering fluids by IV pump or syringe driver

When IV fluids require accurate delivery, IV pumps and syringe drivers are used. Every Trust has a variety of types in use for different purposes (Medical Device Agency 1995):

●   neonatal devices which provide low flow rates in very accurate doses

●   high-risk infusions such as for intravenous drugs, which require pumps to deliver at a set, consistent flow rate with a high degree of accuracy

●   low-risk infusions for routine fluid administration, e.g. through gravity-controlled administration sets where regular delivery is important, but a high level of accuracy is not essential

- patient-controlled analgesia pumps that provides a consistent level of pain relief, with additional bolus doses in response to patient demands
- pre-filled devices that are self-regulating and suitable for care in the community.

Selection of appropriate pump

As technology changes rapidly it is impossible to review all methods here but there are some key considerations to be aware of when caring for a patient with an IV pump. It is important to know why the patient needs an IV pump so that you can select the correct one.

Make sure to check the following issues:

- What is the pump needed for?
- Is it for drug dose accuracy?
- Is it for fast or slow fluid rate?
- Is it because the patient is vulnerable and needs close monitoring? Particular risk factors to be considered are extremes of age (such as the very young or very old), immuno-compromised patients, or cardiac or renal problems.

Preparing to use a pump

If you are unfamiliar with the pumps being used in your location, ask for appropriate training before using one. Be sure you know:

- how to set or change the rate
- how to commence a new infusion
- which administration set is required for each different type in your area
- how to insert the specialist administration set and prime it
- how to respond to the alarm, and reset it
- how to connect the power supply, or switch to battery power. All infusion devices will have a power supply, which is usually backed up by batteries. When not in use most pumps should be kept plugged in to recharge
- how to clean and store it between patients.

Only qualified staff should adjust the rate of flow of an infusion pump as they are held accountable for fluid or drug administration.

ALERT!

Alarms may be muted while dealing with problems, but should never be disabled while the infusion is running, as serious faults may go undetected. If there is a reason to believe the alarm is false, check the entire system including the cannula site. User error may be at fault rather than the machine (Pickstone 1999), so ensure the correct equipment is used, and that the patient's vein is patent. If a thorough check does not reveal the problem, change the pump and seek advice from senior staff.

Gravity infusion sets

These have a flow rate controller integral to the administration set, and there is minimal pressure used to infuse the fluid. To be effective, the IV bag should be raised to at least 1 metre above the patient (Pickstone 1999). Be aware that if the patient is mobilizing and pushing an IV stand around, this distance may not be maintained consistently so will affect the IV flow.

This is not the most accurate method of fluid delivery and so is used for low-risk infusions. It is important to remember the following when using a flow rate controller:

- Calculate the number of drops per minute accurately and monitor it regularly throughout the infusion.
- Explain to the patient that only staff should adjust the rate, and that tampering with the speed may not finish the infusion quicker, but may cause additional problems if fluid is infused too quickly.
- Monitor the amount of fluid that has been infused by observing the level of fluid in the IV bag.
- If the infusion stops or slows, the tubing should *never* be twisted to try to restart the flow. This can cause a high-pressure flow in the vein resulting in spasm, collapse and loss of IV site (Hecker 1988). Ask a qualified nurse to flush the cannula with saline to check the patency instead.

Volumetric pumps

These are used for highly accurate administration of fluids or drugs and use pressure to infuse. Volumes from 1 to 999 ml/hour are delivered depending on the predetermined settings. As well as being able to deliver fluid at a given rate, advancing technology offers additional features, which include:

- running an infusion at 'keep vein open' (KVO) to provide a very slow rate
- monitoring and recording a patient's fluid history
- detecting problems such as air in the administration set or an occlusion in the vein which may trigger the alarm.

It is important to remember the following when using a volumetric pump:

- Use the correct infusion set for the type of machine; otherwise, the infusion can free-flow (Morling 1998).
- Ensure the infusion set is inserted in the machine as outlined in the manufacturer's instructions. No force should be required to insert or remove it.
- Move the tubing in the controller every few hours to prevent compression or tubing damage.

Syringe pumps and drivers

These are used to deliver small amounts of fluid or drugs accurately. Syringe pumps may take 5–60 ml syringes and deliver 0.5–200 ml/hour. Syringe drivers take smaller amounts, up to 35 ml syringes, and deliver in mm/hour rather than ml/hour (Woollon 1997); they therefore need careful calculations to ensure the correct dose is given. Both these devices are usually used in the delivery of complex drug regimes and should be set by a qualified nurse.

It is important to remember the following when caring for a patient with these devices:

- Syringe drivers usually run on batteries, so check the battery indicator regularly to monitor it.
- The cannula site may be intravenous or subcutaneous and should be monitored for any adverse reactions.
- Is it delivering at the correct speed? When receiving a handover

from the previous shift check the position of the syringe then, and check it an hour later to ensure it is running as programmed.

- Continue to observe its progress regularly throughout the shift to ensure that faults can be detected speedily and the patient's drug regime is maintained.

TIP! **There may be a delay between starting the pump and when the drug is actually delivered to the patient. This delay can be avoided by ensuring the syringe is fitted tightly into the pump; ensuring that the 'prime' or 'purge' facility has prepared the tubing and syringe so that it is ready to deliver; or by using a smaller syringe if appropriate (Amoore et al. 2001).**

Evaluation

Mr Elliot's infusion runs according to prescribed schedule.

Intervention: changing an IV solution

- Collect prescribed fluid and check with another nurse against the prescription sheet: Right patient, Right fluid (drug), Right time, Right route, and Right dose.
- Wash hands.
- Open the outer wrapper of the prescribed fluid and check the container for cracks, leaks or breakage in sterility; production date and expiry date; and clear fluid – any discolouration, particles or cloudiness will indicate contamination.
- Invert the bag several times gently, but do not shake to ensure the solution is well mixed. This is particularly important if potassium or other drugs have been added to prevent layers forming (Metheny 1990).
- Take it to the patient and identify him by name, confirming identity with hospital number on wrist band and prescription sheet.
- Place new bag on level surface.
- Turn infusion off by closing the clamp. If an electronic pump is being used stop it.
- Take down the old bag from the IV stand and remove it from the administration set, holding the spike carefully so that it does not touch anything.
- Open the new bag by removing the cap from the port.

- Insert the administration set spike into the port.
- Hang up the bag and ensure fluid is flowing.
- Set the rate or recommence the pump.
- Dispose of bag and wash hands.
- Document on the prescription sheet and fluid balance chart.

Intervention: changing the administration set

Equipment

- IV administration set.
- Gloves.
- Alcohol rub.
- Sterile gauze.
- IV dressing or tape.
- Protective waterproof pad.

Procedure

- Wash hands.
- Gather equipment on a clean tray.
- Go to the patient and confirm his identity. Explain the procedure to gain his consent and cooperation.
- Turn off current infusion.
- Remove the tape that is securing the administration set to the limb and place a waterproof sheet under the patient's arm to protect the bed linen and provide a clean working area. Place the gauze next to the cannula/administration set connection to soak up any fluid leaks.
- Open the new administration set and close the clamp on it.
- Disconnect the old set from the bag, and position it above the patient's heart level.

TIP! **If long enough, the old set can be looped over the IV pole to prevent it from being contaminated or being at a low level.**

- Connect the new set into the bag, squeeze the chamber to half full and run through with fluid, excluding air bubbles (see 'Commencing intravenous therapy', page 144), and hang up the bag. Clip the end of the administration set into the roller clamp.

- Clean hands with alcohol rub and put on gloves.
- Holding the new tubing in your non-dominant hand for easy access, press a finger of your non-dominant hand over the cannulated vein to prevent bleeding (Figure 7.7) and carefully disconnect the old administration set, taking care not to dislodge the cannula.

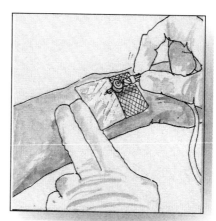

Figure 7.7
Applying pressure to vein above cannula.

WARNING!

The connection may be difficult to twist open. You may see small artery forceps being used to hold the cannula hub to enable disconnection, but this may damage the cannula hub, so use this method with caution.

- Remove the protective cap from the new tubing and connect tubing to the cannula.
- Release pressure from finger on cannula.
- Recommence fluid flow to check for patency, supporting the cannula so that it does not slip out. If in any doubt, get a qualified nurse to flush the cannula with 0.9% saline flush.
- Retape/redress the cannula hub and IV administration set to secure it (Figures 7.4 and 7.5 on pages 148 and 149), wiping around the cannula site with the sterile gauze to remove any leakage during reconnection.

- Set rate of IV flow.
- Label the tubing with date, time of change and your initials.
- Document the change in the nursing notes and fluid balance chart.

NURSING PROBLEM 7.4

Problem: Mr Elliot has an intravenous infusion in situ, and requires daily maintenance of cannula site and infusion to prevent complications of IVT.

Goal: Mr Elliot will not develop any complications of IVT.

Intervention: care of IV infusion and site

- Wash hands. To prevent complications of IV therapy any manipulation of the cannula site or infusion equipment should be undertaken using aseptic principles.
- Check infusion site: (a) before and after commencing a new infusion fluid; (b) when assisting Mr Elliot to wash or dress; (c) before and during IV drug administration; (d) when checking flow rate.
- Observe for: (a) swelling and colour of limb or around cannula entry site: this may indicate infiltration or extravasation; (b) evidence and extent of inflammation, redness or pain: this may suggest phlebitis, infection or nerve injury; (c) leakage from cannula site, slowing or stopping of infusion flow: this may indicate a blocked cannula, possibly from venospasm or infiltration, and may occur especially at night (Campbell 1997); (d) secure dressing or taping of the cannula: if loose, this allows the cannula to move and irritate the vein and may lead to phlebitis; (e) correct rate of fluid delivery: too much may lead to fluid overload, or if it contains a drug may lead to speedshock.
- If any of these are present, stop the infusion and report to senior staff. If the cannula is loose, provided there are no local signs of inflammation or infection it may be secured and redressed following aseptic principles. (See 'Commencing intravenous therapy', page 150.)

- If an infusion has been discontinued, but the cannula not removed immediately, ensure it is removed within 48–72 hours of insertion to prevent complications developing.
- Document your findings and actions. Ensure you have informed a senior nurse or medical staff of any abnormalities.

TIP! **When helping a patient with an IV infusion to dress, thread the infusion set through the sleeve and then put the affected arm in first. To undress, take the arm with the administration set out last and thread the set through the sleeve. This allows the patient more freedom of movement. IVIs should never be disconnected for dressing as it increases the infection risks.**

Summary of IV complications

Local complications

Infiltration

Also known as tissuing. Fluid no longer enters the vein, because either the cannula has slipped out of the vein or the vein has collapsed, causing a blockage and backflow of fluid into the interstitial spaces (Hecker 1988).

Signs/symptoms: Swelling, cool blanched skin, leakage from cannula, infusion slow or stopped, loose cannula.

Interventions: Discontinue IV, elevate arm on pillows or a sling, monitor limb for circulation, motor and sensation. Advise patient that the swelling will recede slowly.

Extravasation

This is when vesicant (toxic) drugs, e.g. 10% or 20% dextrose, or cytotoxic drugs have infiltrated the tissues rather than isotonic fluid, and cause tissue damage (Lamb 1996).

Signs/symptoms: As above, but swelling may be rapid and related to an IV drug injection. There may be some discolouration of the skin.

Interventions: As above, but follow local protocol to provide antidote or hydrocortisone injection. Extravasation can result in tissue necrosis if not corrected quickly.

Phlebitis

The inner lining of the vein is irritated by:

- a chemical such as a drug, or acidic infusion such as potassium chloride
- a physical irritation from the type of cannula used
- the poor placement of a cannula
- mechanical irritation from poor fixation.

Once inflamed the vein may then become infected.

Signs/symptoms: Swelling, inflammation, red, tense and hard vein (induration), possibly purulent discharge at cannula exit site.

Interventions: Discontinue IV, send the cannula for Microscopy Culture and Sensitivity. Use smallest possible cannula to reduce local irritation. Prevention includes careful aseptic site preparation and sterile dressing. Change cannula, dressing and administration set every 48–72 hours. Monitor temperature and pulse every 4 hours for early detection.

Thrombophlebitis

This is when a thrombus (blood clot) forms inside the inflamed vein.

Signs/symptoms: Severe discomfort, inflammation visibly tracking up vein, pyrexia, tachycardia, enlarged lymph glands, raised white cell count.

Interventions: As above, discontinue IV. May need resiting for IV antibiotics. Assess wound for appropriate dressing.

Nerve injury

This may result from the swelling caused by infiltration or extravasation, poor location of cannula, too many attempts at cannulation, or bandaging or splinting too tightly or in an abnormal position (Masoorli 1995; Dougherty 1996).

Signs/symptoms: Pain in hand or arm before and after discontinuation of IV, numbness, tingling.

Interventions: Early detection of infiltration/extravasation and appropriate treatment. If patient complains of pain or discomfort in hand during infusion, report it to a senior member of staff and document it. Check for swelling or inflammation. Discontinue IV. If IVT is continued it should be recommenced on the other limb.

Systemic complications

Bacteraemia

Micro-organisms in the blood. May go undetected until septicaemia develops.

Septicaemia

Presence of pathogenic bacterial toxins in the blood.

Signs/symptoms: General malaise, pyrexia, rigors, nausea, vomiting and hypotension (Lamb 1996). May have evidence of inflammation at cannula site and along the vein, but may be no visible inflammation.

Interventions: Notify the doctor. Take vital signs. Prevention requires maintenance of scrupulous aseptic technique whenever manipulating the IV equipment. Always wash hands before and after touching the system. Keep the number of extensions and three-way taps to the minimum. Change whole system every 48–72 hours. Monitor cannula site for signs of infection. Blood cultures taken and the cannula tip should be sent for microscopy, sensitivity and culture. IV antibiotics and additional therapeutic interventions will be required.

Emboli

Air, particle, catheter or thrombus; occurs when a foreign body enters the circulation and travels until it occludes a small vessel:

● Air embolism may result from poor connections or air bubbles in the IV system.
● Particulate embolism may result from poorly dissolved drug components, or contamination of fluid.

- A catheter emboli may occur either during cannulation if the needle is inadvertently reinserted through the cannula, severing it, or if scissors are used to remove tape, and cut the cannula by accident.
- A thrombus may form inside a vein or on the end of a cannula, and be dislodged when the cannula is flushed.

Signs/symptoms: Breathlessness, chest pain, weak pulse, loss of consciousness. Air noted in administration set. If the cannula is severed the end may be visible.

Interventions: Stop IV. Call for assistance. Take vital signs. Turn patient onto left-hand side to encourage air to rise into the right atrium. If cannula end is visible attempt to retrieve it.

Circulatory overload

This can occur when too much fluid has been infused and the patient is not able to disperse it naturally. It may happen due to a fault in an IV pump or administration set, or positional cannula, or due to over-transfusion.

Signs/symptoms: Discomfort, neck vein enlargement, respiratory distress, cough with white or pink frothy sputum.

Interventions: Stop IV. Inform the doctor. Sit patient up and administer oxygen if prescribed. Ensure patients at risk (see 'Fluid delivery by IV pump', page 154) have fluids administered by pump and check flow rate regularly. Diuretics may be given to increase the rate of fluid excretion.

Drug incompatibility

Patients who are receiving IV drugs may be prescribed drugs that are incompatible with each other, which if administered through the same or connecting IV administration sets may result in a chemical reaction causing particles to form in the infusion.

Signs/symptoms: Blocked cannula, poor infusion flow, evidence of particles in infusion fluid, patient discomfort.

Interventions: Stop infusion, change administration set. Prevent by checking drug compatibility before administration. Inform medical staff.

Speedshock

Caused by the rapid infusion of an IV drug resulting in a toxic blood concentration.

Signs/symptoms: Flushed face, headache, dizziness, chest tightness, tachycardia and hypotension.

Interventions: Stop infusion. Provide symptomatic relief, e.g. sitting up, oxygen therapy. Take vital signs. May need to be given an antidote. Inform medical staff. Prevent by administering through a pump, burette or by syringe driver.

Anaphylactic/allergic reaction

This is a result of allergen or drug reaction and can be very sudden and life-threatening.

Signs/symptoms: Itching, rash, watering eyes, sneezing, bronchospasm, facial flushing, and swelling, anxiety, rapid swelling at IV site, sudden collapse, cardiac arrest.

Interventions: Discontinue infusion immediately. Call for urgent assistance. Take vital signs. Maintain airway. Administer epinephrine according to local policy. Prevent by taking a thorough history of allergy, and monitor patient closely when giving potential allergens.

Removal of cannulas

Cannulas should be removed as soon as possible after therapy has been discontinued (Spencer 1996), otherwise patients could be exposed to unnecessary infection risks.

Intervention: removal of IV cannula

Equipment

- Sterile gauze.
- Hypoallergenic tape.
- Gloves.
- Small sharps disposal box.

Procedure

- Wash hands.
- Collect equipment on a clean tray.
- Explain the procedure to Mr Elliot and gain his cooperation. Provide privacy.
- If infusion is still in progress, turn off. Record amount of fluid administered.
- Put on gloves.
- Open gauze swabs.
- Loosen dressing and remove from the skin. An elderly patient's skin may be fragile and tear easily (Whitson 1996), so ease off gently. Observe site for signs of inflammation or infection.
- With your non-dominant hand, put pressure over the end of the cannula in the vein.
- Fold a piece of gauze in half and hold in your non-dominant hand.
- With your dominant hand, withdraw cannula. As soon as it has been removed place the folded gauze on the entry site and apply pressure for 2–3 minutes until bleeding stops.
- Apply a fresh piece of gauze and secure with hypoallergenic tape. If infection or localized tissue damage is present, apply appropriate dressing.
- Dispose of equipment, placing cannula in sharps container.
- Ensure Mr Elliot is comfortable and has all he needs.
- Record removal in the nursing notes, documenting your observations of the condition of the site. Observe the site closely over the next 24 hours to ensure that post-infusion phlebitis does not occur (Millam 1988). If there are no signs of inflammation or infection the dressing can be removed after 8–12 hours, and the site exposed.

Evaluation

Mr Elliot's infusion site heals with no complications or discomfort.

Blood transfusion

The aim of a blood transfusion is to increase the oxygen delivery to the tissues in a short time (Togshill 1997). It is the most effective method of replacing acute blood loss, but whole blood is rarely used as various blood components are extracted and used for a variety of purposes. Blood can be considered as living tissue and as such there are several risks associated with transfusion. Incorrect transfusions have frequently been found to result from errors involving incorrect identity of the patient or of the blood, and there are several stages in the process when these errors can occur (SHOT 1999). To promote safe practice for the care of patients receiving a blood transfusion, national guidelines have been published by the British Committee for Standards in Haematology Blood Transfusion Task Force (BCSH 1999). The prescribing of blood and blood components is the sole responsibility of medical staff unless local guidelines have determined otherwise (BCSH 1999).

Blood products for transfusion

Whole blood

Contents: Red and white blood cells and plasma.

Uses: Replacement of red cells and plasma proteins as in massive blood loss.

Red cells

Contents: Concentrated red cells, reduced plasma component, in additive solution such as saline, adenine, glucose and mannitol (SAG-M).

Uses: To restore oxygen-carrying capacity in chronic or haemolytic anaemia, or replace blood loss.

Platelets

Contents: Concentrated platelets in plasma, with red cells removed.

Uses: To treat clotting abnormalities as a result of large transfusions or thrombocytopenia (too few platelets resulting in haemorrhage).

Fresh frozen plasma

Contents: Plasma and plasma components frozen within eight hours of collection.

Uses: Bleeding disorders where clotting factors are absent.

Patient history

Mr Ammon has been involved in a road traffic accident (RTA) having been knocked off his motor cycle. He has a suspected fractured pelvis, left fractured femur and a right compound fracture of tibia and fibula, and possible internal injuries. It is estimated that he will need at least four units of blood to compensate for the blood loss from the accident and the surgical operation.

NURSING PROBLEM 7.5

Problem: Mr Ammon requires a blood transfusion and is at risk of adverse reactions.

Goal: Prevention and early detection of adverse reactions to blood transfusion.

Preventing adverse reactions to blood transfusions

To minimize risk factors there are some key points where specific safety measures should be adopted:

- blood sample collection for cross-matching
- collection, storage and transport
- checking before administration
- care during administration.

Blood sample collection for cross-matching

To minimize hazards that may result in the wrong blood type being administered to a patient the BCSH (1999) guidelines recommend:

- The patient's identity should be confirmed verbally if possible. If the patient is unconscious additional confirmation using gender and hospital number should be included.
- Identity is confirmed with the identity band giving full name, date of birth, gender and hospital number.

- The request form must include surname, first name, gender, date of birth, hospital number.
- Blood samples should be labelled directly after collection and while beside the patient so that details can be checked immediately. Addressograph labels should not be used on sample tubes.
- Any factors, such as previous transfusions and current medication that may contribute to potential complications should be identified during preliminary nursing and medical assessments for transfusion (Bradbury and Cruickshank 2000).

Collection, storage and transport

Collection of blood for transfusion should only occur when:

- the prescription has been written
- the patient has a patent IV access ready for transfusion
- the patient's consent has been obtained and any concerns that he may have regarding the integrity of the transfusion have been allayed.

Patients may express particular concerns regarding their religious views or the transmission of blood-borne viruses such as HIV, new variant CJD, or hepatitis B or C. Reassurance may be given that all donated blood in the UK is screened for these infective diseases, and that the UK has implemented a process called 'leucocyte depletion' to reduce potential infection and reaction risks (Gray and Murphy 1999). Leucocyte depletion involves the leucocytes being removed from the blood before transfusion to reduce potential reactions and transmission of infection.

Anxieties relating to religious or ethical concerns may be of concern to Mr Ammon so a clear explanation of the benefits and risks of transfusion should be offered to enable him to make an informed decision about his treatment (Atterbury and Wilkinson 2000).

Once blood has been removed from the storage fridge transfusion should commence within 30 minutes. If transfusion does not commence within 30 minutes, blood should *not* be stored in a non-blood fridge, but the blood bank should be contacted to confirm whether it is safe to commence transfusion, or if the unit should be returned to the haematology department. Blood should be used within 4 hours of leaving cold storage (Togshill 1997), since micro-organisms may multiply and the quality of the red cells deteriorate.

To collect a unit from storage (Atterbury and Wilkinson 2000):

● Take the compatibility report (cross-match form) or prescription sheet with the details to the blood bank.
● Check that the blood label on the unit agrees with the patient details: full name, hospital number, date of birth, required blood component, for example red cells or whole blood, and number of units issued.
● Confirm blood group on unit with patient details and compatibility report.
● Select units in order (depending on number required for transfusion), and close door firmly.
● Sign with the date, time and name in the blood bank register.
● Transport to clinical area in bag or tray if provided. Care should be taken not to damage the pack in transit.
● The pack should be delivered directly to the qualified practitioner responsible for administration.

Checking before administration

Equipment required to commence a blood transfusion

● Prescription sheet.
● Compatibility form.
● Fluid balance chart.
● Disinfected tray containing the following:
   – IV cannula; usual size for blood transfusion is 21 gauge (green) or above (19 or 20 gauge).
   – Alcohol wipes or chlorhexidine cleanser.
   – Blood administration set.
   – IV pole/stand.
   – Sterile dressing and tape or semi-permeable transparent IV dressing.
   – Gloves.

IV access

● IV access should be obtained before blood is collected from storage. (See 'Commencing an infusion', page 144.)

This is the final opportunity to detect any errors of incompatibility. Unfortunately failure to follow stringent procedures has resulted in fatalities (Gray and Murphy 1999). The qualified nurse is as accountable for safety during transfusion as during drug administration. As an unqualified practitioner, you may find yourself checking blood with a qualified practitioner, and should remain accountable for your actions. Be vigilant at all stages, even if Trust policy considers the qualified practitioner as ultimately responsible as if administering a drug single-handedly. Blood unit numbers can be long and mistakes can easily be made.

Final checks

All checks should be done at the patient bedside (Gray and Murphy 1999):

- Confirm Mr Ammon's identity, verbally and from his wrist band. Check first name and surname, date of birth, gender and hospital number.
- Check identity details on blood compatibility form and confirm against identity wrist band.
- Confirm compatibility between blood unit number, type and blood compatibility form with the label on the blood pack (Figure 7.8).

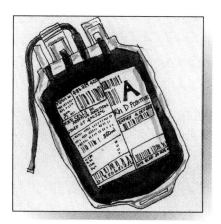

Figure 7.8
Blood unit details.

- Confirm patient identity and blood request with the prescription form and medical notes.
- Check the blood bag for expiry date, possible leaks around seams or entry points. Look for any abnormal presentation of contents such as air bubbles, discolouration or clotting (Bradbury and Cruickshank 2000).
- Check the prescription sheet for any medication required prior to or during the infusion.
- If all checks tally proceed to transfusion.

ALERT!

The blood group ABO and Rhesus factor on the blood unit and compatibility form should be identical. In cases of emergency transfusion, O Rhesus negative may be used as it is the universal donor (Table 7.1). If there is any doubt or discrepancy between the group on the blood unit and the blood group of the patient, contact the blood bank immediately and do not commence the infusion.

No drugs should be added to the blood or administration set as they could contaminate or react with the blood. If intravenous drugs are required ensure that the patient has two patent IV access sites, or a Y type cannula may be used, depending on local policy.

Approximately 85 per cent of people in the UK are Rhesus D positive. Those who are Rh D negative have no Rhesus antigen, but a Rh D antibody can be produced after exposure to Rh D positive blood (Glover and Powell 1996). This will have consequences for the recipient so check that the Rh D is compatible.

Table 7.1 Blood group compatibility

Blood group	Compatible groups	Percentage in UK
O	O	47 (O Rh −ve = universal donor)
A	A and O	42
B	B and O	8
AB	AB, A, B, and O	3 (AB Rh +ve = universal recipient)

Care during administration

Close monitoring of the patient during blood administration will detect any adverse reactions.

Intervention: safe blood transfusion

- Take baseline vital signs of temperature, pulse and respiratory rate (TPR), and BP and commence an observation record solely for the period of transfusion.
- Ensure a blood administration set with an integral filter is ready for use. An IV administration set may be primed with 0.9% saline solution before transfusion, but Atterbury and Wilkinson (2000) suggest that this may prevent complete filling with blood and some filters and administration sets should not be primed in this way. Alternatively, the IV cannula can have patency confirmed with a 0.9% saline flush and the blood administration set primed then with blood. The drip and filter chambers should be filled half full before the tubing clamp is opened and the tubing filled, to exclude as much air as possible so that blood is not wasted. (To prepare an infusion see 'Commencing an IV', page 144.)

ALERT!

Only 0.9% saline solutions should come into contact with blood or blood products. If dextrose is given it will cause haemolysis (breakdown of red blood cells).

- Set the rate of flow as calculated.
- A severe reaction may commence within the first 10–15 minutes of infusion as it takes very little incompatible blood to cause a reaction (Bradbury and Cruickshank 2000). The patient should be in a position for close observation during transfusion. Some Trusts require a nurse to remain present during the first 10–15 minutes. Research evidence has not yet identified the ideal frequency to monitor vital signs but Gray and Murphy (1999) and Bradbury and Cruickshank (2000) suggest that TPR and BP should be recorded:

- before the transfusion begins
- 15 minutes after commencement of each unit
- temperature and pulse may be recorded more regularly during transfusion, e.g. every 15 minutes of the first hour and hourly thereafter
- on completion of the transfusion
- 4-hourly for 24 hours after completion to identify any post-transfusion reaction.

TIP! Unconscious patients should have hourly observations throughout a transfusion as they are unable to communicate any discomfort. Observe urine output closely for any signs of haematuria (blood).

- Mr Ammon should be advised to report any feelings of breathlessness, loin pain, abdominal discomfort, shivering, or feeling unwell. He should be observed for pyrexia, tachycardia, rashes, flushing or blood in his urine. If any of these occur stop the transfusion and seek medical advice.
- Documentation of vital signs and blood pack details should be completed and maintained throughout the treatment. Should any adverse reactions occur (see section below) inform senior nurse and medical staff. Document your response and interventions in the nursing record.
- A permanent record of the following should be kept in the medical notes (Gray and Murphy 1999):
  - type of transfusion of blood or blood products
  - compatibility form
  - nursing observation record
  - indications for and response to the transfusion
  - occurrence and management of adverse reactions.
- A fluid balance record should be maintained, recording the amount of each unit, the patient's overall fluid balance and if blood was detected in the urine during transfusion.
- On completion the blood bag is sealed with the attached bung, placed in an outer bag, and discarded or returned to the haematology department, depending on the local policy. A new administration set should be used for any subsequent fluids, or the cannula may be removed.

Evaluation

Mr Ammon receives a blood transfusion without adverse reactions.

Common adverse reactions

Pyrexia

Mild: Up to 38°C.

Actions: Stop or slow transfusion; inform medical staff; administer paracetamol and observe response to medication.

Severe: Temperature above 38°C, rigors/shivering.

Actions: Stop infusion; inform medical staff; maintain IV access with 0.9% saline via new administration set; administer antipyretics as prescribed.

Allergic reaction

Mild: Urticarial rash (hives), pyrexia.

Severe: Facial oedema, bronchospasm.

Actions: Stop infusion; administer antihistamines. In case of a severe reaction respond as for an emergency.

Infections

Symptoms: Pyrexia, rigors, hypotension, phlebitis at IV site.

Actions: Stop infusion. Inform medical staff. Save unit of blood and return to blood bank for analysis.

Haemolytic reaction

Symptoms: Destruction of donor red cells by recipient causing: pain at IV site; facial flushing; back or loin pain; falling BP and raised temperature and pulse; decreased urine output; blood in urine; breathlessness; collapse. This can be severe and is life-threatening.

Actions: Stop transfusion immediately; take vital signs; maintain IV access with 0.9% saline solution. Inform medical staff urgently.

Circulatory overload

Symptoms: Breathlessness; cough; distress.

Actions: Stop or slow infusion; diuretic therapy; monitor urine output.

TIP! Emergency drugs such as IM epinephrine and IV piriton should be readily available when blood transfusions are in progress in case of allergic reaction.

Further reading

Amoore J, Dewar D, Ingram P, Lowe D (2001) Syringe pumps and start up time: ensuring safe practice. Nursing Standard 15(17): 43–45.

Bradbury M, Cruickshank JL (2000) Blood transfusion: crucial steps in maintaining safe practice. British Journal of Nursing 9(3): 134–38.

Morling S (1998) Infusion devices: risks and user responsibilities. British Journal of Nursing 7(1): 13–19.

Woollon S (1997) Selection of intravenous and infusion pumps. Professional Nurse Supplement 12(8): S14–S15.

Workman B (1999) Peripheral intravenous therapy management. Nursing Standard 14(4): 53–60.

CHAPTER 8

Respiratory care

Clare Bennett

Aims and learning outcomes

This chapter introduces the fundamental principles of respiratory assessment and symptom management. By the end of the chapter you should be able to:

- carry out fundamental aspects of respiratory assessment, including the following: obtain a patient's history; make observations of respiratory rate, depth and rhythm, cyanosis and sputum; record peak expiratory flow rate and pulse oximetry
- administer oxygen safely
- administer nebulizer therapy
- describe the general principles of correct inhaler technique
- perform oropharyngeal and nasopharyngeal suctioning.

Respiratory assessment

The respiratory tract is made up of the nose, pharynx, larynx, trachea, bronchi and lungs. A problem arising in any part of the tract may result in breathlessness. Additionally, disturbances in the circulatory, haematological and metabolic systems have the potential to affect normal respiratory patterns.

Respiratory assessment begins with observing a patient's general appearance. Factors to observe include:

- Facial expression – does the patient appear alert, orientated, exhausted, confused, anxious or unresponsive? Are there any non-verbal expressions of pain, for example, grimaces, facial distortion, lip biting? Is there any evidence of facial flushing or cyanosis?
- Posture – is the patient sitting erect, or in a slouched or crouched-forward posture? Does the posture suggest pain in a particular place? Does the posture indicate anxiety or fear? Does the patient suffer from orthopnoea (i.e. breathlessness when lying down)?
- Physical symptoms – can the patient talk in full sentences or is breathlessness only upon exertion? Is there an increase in chest size (barrel-chested), coughing, or production of sputum?

The second aspect of respiratory assessment requires information from the patient concerning his symptoms, their onset and his past medical and social history. It is necessary to know:

- the nature and severity of symptoms (e.g. breathlessness, increased sputum production, pain, cough, fever)
- precipitating factors such as exposure to infection, smoking, known allergies and exposure to irritants
- duration of symptoms
- past medical history related to breathing difficulties
- general health status
- medications taken
- psychosocial history, including age, occupational history, information concerning the patient's living conditions and the patient's perception of the illness.

TIP! When gathering information from an acutely breathless patient, use short questions that can be answered 'Yes' or 'No'. These are called 'closed' questions. The patient may not have enough breath to talk in sentences. Look in the notes for extra information to avoid wearing the patient out with repeated questions that other staff have already asked.

The third aspect of respiratory assessment uses physical examination and observations. These will be explained in the following nursing interventions. The specific values and times have not been included as every patient will have slightly different needs when considering frequency of observations.

Normal values

Normal respiratory values will vary according to a patient's age, gender and medical history. The normal rate of breathing at rest is 12–20 times per minute for a healthy adult.

Terminology

apnoea	when there is no breathing; periods of apnoea may be interspersed with bradypnoea
bradypnoea	abnormally slow rate of breathing (less than 12 breaths per minute); possible causes include hypothermia and depression of the central nervous system
dyspnoea	difficult, laboured or uncomfortable breathing
hyperpnoea	an increase in the volume of air breathed per minute; this is caused by an increase in the depth and/or respiratory rate
tachypnoea	an abnormally fast rate of breathing (more than 20 breaths per minute); this is usually one of the first signs of respiratory distress

---

Normal breathing

On inspiration the diaphragm descends, the lower part of the rib cage moves upward and outward and there is slight expansion of the upper chest. Expiration is passive and is slightly longer than inspiration. A short pause is normal between expiration and the next inspiration. Chest movement should be equal, bilateral and symmetrical. It is important to monitor the respiratory rate, rhythm and depth of any patient who has an altered respiratory status.

Normal breathing should be barely audible to the naked ear, but with a stethoscope will be equal on both sides and audible in all the lung zones. The following sounds are significant:

● Noisy respiration is a sign of respiratory distress.

- Stridor is a high-pitched sound usually occurring on inspiration; it is caused by laryngeal or tracheal obstruction, such as tumour or foreign body.
- A 'wheeze' is characterized by a noisy musical sound caused by the turbulent flow of air through narrowed bronchi and bronchioles (Jevon and Ewens 2001). A 'wheeze' is often more pronounced on expiration and is associated with asthma, chronic bronchitis and emphysema.
- A 'rattly chest' is caused by the presence of fluid (pulmonary oedema or sputum) in the upper airway.
- Snoring sounds, in the unconscious patient, may be associated with the tongue blocking the airway.

NURSING PROBLEM 8.1

Patient history: Mr Brown has been admitted to the ward with breathlessness and a productive cough.

Problem: Mr Brown's respirations are rapid and irregular (30 breaths per minute).

Goal: Mr Brown's respirations will return to normal parameters (x breaths per minute) within y hours of admission.

TIP! When observing an individual's respiratory rate, rhythm and depth it is advisable not to let the patient know you are doing this, since people tend to breathe differently if they know someone is watching. It is therefore a good idea to make these observations immediately after taking the pulse. As you are continuing to hold the patient's wrist he will not be aware that you are actually observing his respirations.

Intervention: measuring respiratory rate

The most sensitive indicator of respiratory distress is a rise in an individual's respiratory rate (Hinds and Watson 1996).

- Ensure that Mr Brown has been at rest for approximately five minutes.
- Continue to hold the wrist you used to take Mr Brown's pulse and watch his chest rise and fall.
- Look at your watch and count the number of times the chest rises in 60 seconds. This is Mr Brown's respiratory rate, measured as 'breaths per minute'.
- Record the measurement on Mr Brown's observations chart and inform a senior member of staff in the event of any change in respiratory rate.

TIP! If the patient's breathing is very shallow and therefore difficult to see, place your hand on the patient's chest or abdomen to feel for movement. Count the number of times your hand rises in 60 seconds. This is the patient's respiratory rate, measured as 'breaths per minute'.

Intervention: observing respiratory rhythm

Normal breathing is regular and rhythmic. When measuring respiratory rate observe the pattern of breathing and its regularity. For example, the 'Cheyne-Stokes' pattern of breathing is characterized by periods of apnoea alternated with periods of increasingly rapid and deep breathing. This often occurs in patients nearing the end of life. 'Kussmaul' breathing is characterized by deep rapid respirations triggered by stimulation of the respiratory centres in the medulla and pons of the brainstem, caused by metabolic acidosis and is a result of renal failure or diabetic ketoacidosis.

Intervention: monitoring respiratory depth

Air entry is assessed through observing and feeling chest movements in addition to listening to breath sounds.

- Observe Mr Brown for use of the accessory muscles of ventilation. These are to be seen in the neck, upper chest and abdomen (sternocleidomastoid, trapezius and pectoral muscles). In adults, the use of these accessory muscles suggests respiratory distress. In the elderly, abdominal breathing is considered normal. If the patient is using these muscles, it should be reported and documented.

- 'Ballooning out' of the intercostal spaces (i.e. the spaces between the ribs) during exhalation or retraction during inspiration should be documented and reported.
- Your observations of Mr Brown's respiratory depth should be documented and a senior member of staff should be informed of any changes.

Intervention: measuring effectiveness of respiration

Observe for evidence of cyanosis (blue tinge to the skin).

Normal saturated haemoglobin gives mucous membranes their characteristic pink colour. Unsaturated haemoglobin gives mucous membranes a bluish/purple discoloration. Cyanosis is associated with excessive deoxygenation of haemoglobin and hypoxia. It is therefore characterized by a dusky bluish colour of the mucous membranes.

Peripheral cyanosis is observed in the skin and nail beds and is most noticeable around the lips, earlobes, mouth and fingertips. In dark-skinned people cyanosis is most noticeable in the lips or nailbeds, which become dusky in colour. Peripheral cyanosis alone suggests circulatory problems rather than respiratory disease.

Central cyanosis is best observed in the tongue; it may be an acute sign of hypoxia (e.g. asphyxia) or a chronic sign of respiratory disease (e.g. chronic obstructive pulmonary disease).

Your assessment and findings regarding any peripheral and central cyanosis should be documented in Mr Brown's notes and communicated to a senior member of staff.

Intervention: measuring pulse oximetry

Assessing the amount of oxygen absorbed in the arterial blood will give an indication of the effectiveness of the patient's breathing and/or oxygen therapy. This can be done by using pulse oximetry. A two-sided probe is used to transmit an alternating light through a finger, toe or earlobe. The wavelength of the light that emerges indicates the percentage of oxyhaemoglobin present in the capillaries (Woodrow 1999).

Normal values of oxygen saturation are 95–99%. Readings of 90–95% are usually a cause for concern. However, the patient's medical history must be taken into consideration when interpreting readings; for example, a patient with chronic obstructive pulmonary disease may usually have an oxygen saturation of 85% (Woodrow 1999).

TIP! When monitoring a patient's pulse oximetry, don't rely exclusively on the pulse oximeter recording to tell you if the patient is receiving adequate ventilation. Watch for signs of respiratory distress and changes in skin colour too.

Equipment

- Pulse oximeter.
- Appropriate sensor.
- Trolley/table to mount monitor on.

Procedure

- Explain the procedure to Mr Brown to gain his consent and co-operation.
- Assess Mr Brown's peripheral circulation in order to select an appropriate sensor. The most commonly used sensor is a finger sensor, but others are available that can be attached to the earlobe and external nose.
- Clean the skin and dry the area thoroughly. If using a finger sensor, false nails and nail polish should be removed to prevent an inaccurate reading.
- Attach the sensor according to the manufacturer's instructions, attach the cable from the sensor to the pulse oximeter and switch the machine on.
- Observe the pulse waveform or digital readout to ensure that the pulse waveform is registering.
- Set alarm limits on the pulse oximeter.
- Change the sensor site every 4 hours if continuous monitoring is required, in order to relieve pressure and any irritation from adhesive sensors. If intermittent monitoring is required remove the sensor between readings.
- Document Mr Brown's oxygen saturation in the nursing records and report any changes or abnormal readings immediately.

ALERT!

Never attach a finger sensor by using adhesive tape, since this has the potential to cause tissue necrosis.

Intervention: recording peak expiratory flow rate (PEFR)

The peak expiratory flow rate (PEFR) is a measurement of the maximum flow rate, in litres per minute, that can be expelled from the lungs during a forced exhalation. Measuring PEFR indicates how severe the patient's airway obstruction may be.

Equipment

- Peak flow meter (Figure 8.1).
- Disposable mouthpiece.
- Recording chart.

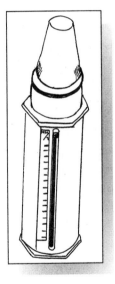

Figure 8.1
The Mini-Wright peak flow meter.

Procedure

- Explain the procedure to Mr Brown to gain his cooperation.
- Advise Mr Brown to stand; if this is not possible, he should sit as upright as possible to allow for maximum lung expansion.
- Attach the disposable mouthpiece to the peak flow meter.
- Place the cursor at the bottom of the numbered scale.
- Advise Mr Brown to inhale as deeply as possible, to place his lips around the mouthpiece creating a complete seal, and hold the meter horizontally to exhale as hard and fast as possible, as if blowing out a candle.

- Note the measurement obtained.
- Ask Mr Brown to repeat this process two more times, as long as this does not cause distress. If it is not possible for him to obtain further measurements document this on the observations chart.

TIP! If Mr Brown is very breathless and his second peak flow level is less than the first, don't ask him to do it a third time as he may develop bronchospasm. Seek medical advice.

- Record the highest of three measurements; by having three attempts poor technique should be overcome.
- Report any variation from previous readings to a senior colleague.

TIP! To ensure you get the best reading in a PEFR:

get a good seal between the patient's lips and the mouthpiece zero the meter before blowing
keep fingers out of the way of the measurement indicator.

Intervention: making regular observations of temperature, blood pressure and heart rate

It is important to monitor a breathless patient's vital signs in order to exclude or identify underlying causes of breathlessness. The breathless patient will initially exhibit tachycardia; however, severe hypoxia can lead to bradycardia.

Measurement of temperature, blood pressure and heart rate is detailed in Chapter 2.

TIP! ECG monitoring may be required for some breathless patients. Additional training and skills are needed to per-form ECG monitoring effectively.

Intervention: observation of cough and production of sputum

The assessment of Mr Brown's cough includes observation of the following characteristics:

- frequency
- length of time coughing takes

- presence or absence of pain
- distinctive sounds (e.g. whoop or bark)
- strength of cough
- any association with specific activities (e.g. after eating or drinking).

These observations should be noted in Mr Brown's notes and communicated to other members of the care team.

Intervention: positioning to assist breathing

- Position Mr Brown in an upright position, well supported with pillows. People who are feeling breathless tend to be more comfortable, and respiratory function is maximized, in this position.
- Breathless patients may find sitting in a chair more comfortable than lying in bed.
- Chronically breathless patients may be reluctant to change position frequently and therefore it is important to provide pressure-relieving aids for the sacrum and heels.
- Mr Brown may appreciate a bed table with a pillow on it, placed in front of him so that he can lean forward to aid lung expansion.
- A fan may be positioned to 'blow' over Mr Brown to give him the sensation of more circulating air. This can provide psychological relief.

Intervention: administering oxygen

The administration of oxygen is used to increase the saturation of the oxyhaemoglobin in the blood to compensate for hypoxia.

ALERT!

When administering oxygen it is essential that the following precautions are observed to prevent fire:

Smoking in the area is prohibited.

Signs regarding the prohibition of smoking are displayed.

Matches and lighters should be removed from the patient's bedside.

The use of oil- and alcohol-based skincare products is avoided.

To administer oxygen an oxygen delivery system is required. This consists of:

- An oxygen supply: this may provided through oxygen ports on the walls of hospital wards or via portable cylinders which are coloured black with a white top and marked 'oxygen'.
- Flow meter: this allows the flow rate of oxygen to be set in litres/ minute.
- Oxygen tubing: this connects the oxygen source to the delivery device.
- Delivery device: there are various methods of oxygen delivery. These may provide either a variable concentration of oxygen, or a fixed, accurate concentration. These are termed *variable* or *fixed performance devices* respectively (see below). The device used should reflect the individual patient's oxygen requirements, as well as his comfort and individual choice.

ALERT!

Oxygen should always be prescribed by a doctor, stating the flow rate, delivery system, duration and monitoring of treatment.

- Humidifier: humidification is recommended for patients who receive flow rates of oxygen which are greater than 4 litres per minute, or when oxygen is being delivered directly to the trachea, for example, via a tracheostomy tube (Jevon and Ewens, 2001). Humidification warms and moistens the oxygen during administration, thus preventing dehydration of the mucous membranes and pulmonary secretions (see below).

Fixed performance devices

If a fixed performance device is required, systems such as Venturi devices (Figure 8.2) may be used. These systems allow:

- Specific levels of air entry so that air is mixed with the oxygen administered, to deliver precisely controlled percentages of high flow oxygen at low to mid concentration (24–60 per cent).
- The valves are colour coded according to the percentage of

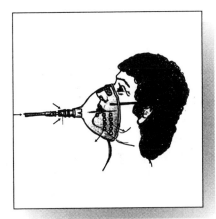

Figure 8.2
Venturi mask.

oxygen delivered. These masks are particularly useful when it is important to administer accurate concentrations of oxygen, for example, in patients with chronic obstructive pulmonary disease.

Other fixed performance devices include continuous positive airway pressure (CPAP) and non-rebreathable masks.

Variable performance devices

If variable performance devices are acceptable, Hudson oxygen masks (Figure 8.3.1) or nasal cannulas may be used (Figure 8.3.2).

These devices deliver an unpredictable oxygen concentration, determined by the patient's respiratory pattern; they are therefore not suitable for patients with chronic respiratory disease.

Nasal cannulae are of limited use for the extremely breathless patient who mouth breathes since the concentration of oxygen will be further diluted (Dunn and Chrisholm 1998). However, nasal cannulae are highly appropriate when patients cannot tolerate face masks.

Humidification devices

Humidification devices vary between Trusts and include:

- aerosol generators
- humidified ventimask systems
- condensers
- water bath humidifiers.

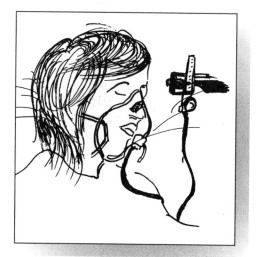

Figure 8.3.1
Hudson mask.

Figure 8.3.2
Nasal cannula.

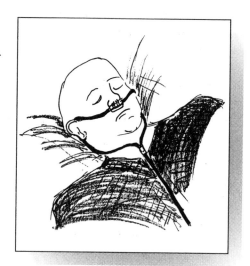

Figure 8.3.1–2 Variable performance devices.

TIP! If using warm humidification, water will collect in the wide-bore 'elephant' tubing. This should be emptied by turning off the oxygen, disconnecting the tubing from the humidifier, pouring the water into a receiver, and reconnecting the tubing and re-commencing oxygen therapy. Water will empty out more easily if the tube is slightly stretched and shaken when emptied.

Intervention: administering medication as prescribed

Depending upon the cause of breathlessness, medications may include:

- bronchodilators (inhaled, nebulized or intravenous)
- intramuscular adrenaline
- intravenous antibiotics
- steroids (nebulized, inhaled or intravenous).

Chapter 6 explains the principles of medicine administration. Mrs Jones's care plan later in this chapter outlines the administration of nebulizers and inhalers.

Intervention: explaining all procedures and the plan of care to Mr Brown

Breathlessness is an extremely frightening experience that often leads to anxiety, which may be aggravated by hypoxia. Anxiety may, in turn, contribute further to Mr Brown's dyspnoea. Discussing with Mr Brown and his family and the provision of information concerning the disease/illness, its management and the plan of care may relieve these common worries. Privacy should be provided and the relatives involved in his care. Relaxation and breathing techniques to improve lung expansion may also be of value.

Intervention: administering oxygen as prescribed

Equipment

- Nasal cannulae or appropriate face mask.
- Oxygen tubing.
- Humidifier.
- Oxygen source with flow meter.
- 'No Smoking' signs.

Procedure

- Check prescription for accuracy.
- Explain the procedure to Mr Brown to reduce his anxiety and gain consent.

- Wash hands and dry thoroughly.
- Prepare equipment.
- Explain the dangers of smoking when oxygen is in use to Mr Brown and his visitors and relatives.
- Check Mr Brown's identity band.
- Attach the oxygen tubing to the oxygen supply and the delivery device (mask or nasal cannulae).
- Turn on the oxygen flow meter and set the prescribed flow rate.
- Ensure that Mr Brown is positioned upright, if possible, to maximize lung expansion.
- If using a face mask, place the mask over Mr Brown's nose and mouth with the elastic strap over the ears to the back of the head. The mask should cover the nose and mouth securely, so it may be necessary to alter the length of elastic.
- If using humidification, connect the humidifier to the oxygen port according to the manufacturer's instructions. Connect wide-bore 'elephant' tubing which comes from the humidifier to the face mask. Set the flow meter as required. Adjust the position of the oxygen mask to cover the nose and mouth securely.
- If using nasal cannulae, the prongs of the cannulae should be placed inside the nostrils and the external tubing should be placed over the ears and either under the chin or behind the head (Figure 8.3.2). The flow rate of oxygen with nasal cannulae must not exceed 4 litres/minute to prevent discomfort and damage to the nasal mucosa (Lifecare 2000).
- Place a sputum pot, tissues and mouthwash near to Mr Brown to use as required.
- Wash hands.
- Document the care given.
- Monitor and record oxygen saturation and respiratory rate, depth and rhythm. Report any abnormalities.

Intervention: comfort measures for patients requiring oxygen therapy

- Assess facial pressure points that contact mask or elastic, nasal cannula (nostrils, external nose and ears) for skin irritation or signs of breakdown every 4 hours. Placing gauze under the elastic may relieve pressure and provide comfort.

- Oral hygiene and oral fluids should be offered frequently to prevent drying of the oral mucosa.
- Cleansing and drying of the face should be offered as required.
- Oxygen tubing and delivery devices should be labelled with the patient's name and hospital number to prevent patient's equipment being used by others in error. This will help to reduce the risk of cross-infection.

TIP! If using an oxygen cylinder, ensure that a replacement cylinder is available when the volume gauge indicates that the cylinder is a quarter full.

TIP! If the patient has to leave the ward for investigations, ensure that the portable oxygen cylinder is full and that the department the patient is visiting knows that continuous oxygen will be required.

ALERT!

The administration of oxygen, except in a very low concentration (24–28 per cent), could be fatal to patients with chronic pulmonary disease. This is because carbon dioxide is retained in the blood (chronic hypercapnia) and the chemoreceptors in the brain become less sensitive to high blood levels of carbon dioxide. The patient then becomes dependent on low oxygen (hypoxia) to stimulate respiration. Thus if oxygen is given to correct hypoxia, the patient's respiratory drive may be removed.

Intervention: observing and collecting sputum

Observe quantity and nature of sputum and obtain a sputum specimen for microscopy, culture and sensitivity.

Sputum is a clinical feature of respiratory disease and can provide valuable information for assessing a breathless patient. Sputum should be observed for consistency, colour and quantity. Patients may refer to it as phlegm.

Thick, viscid sputum is an indication of severe asthma. Thin, watery sputum is a feature of acute pulmonary oedema. White mucoid sputum is characteristic of asthma and chronic bronchitis. Purulent green or yellow sputum may suggest respiratory infection. Blood may indicate carcinoma of the lung or pulmonary embolism. Foul smelling sputum is suggestive of a respiratory tract infection (Jevon and Ewens 2001).

Equipment

- Universal specimen pot.
- Specimen bag.
- Laboratory request form.
- Mouthwash.
- Receiver.
- Tissues.
- Handwashing facilities.

Procedure

- Prepare equipment.
- Encourage Mr Brown to sit upright and take some deep breaths.
- Ask Mr Brown to cough and expectorate into the specimen container. Several coughs may be required to obtain a sufficient specimen. Some patients may need to be taught by a physiotherapist how to cough effectively and expectorate without strain.
- Seal the lid and complete Mr Brown's details on the specimen pot.
- Place pot and laboratory request form in a plastic specimen bag and send to the appropriate laboratory. Wash hands. If a delay in transporting the specimen to the laboratory is envisaged place it in the refrigerator immediately.
- Offer the patient a mouthwash and tissues.
- Document that a specimen has been obtained, noting colour, smell and consistency.

TIP! **Mr Brown may find it easier to produce a specimen on waking up in the morning as he may have more energy for deep coughing and sputum may have settled in the upper lobes of his lungs overnight.**

Evaluation

Has Mr Brown's respiration reverted to its normal rate, rhythm and depth? Has his colour and perfusion improved? If Mr Brown's respiration has not returned to its normal pattern within the stated time the plan of care will need to be revised accordingly.

NURSING PROBLEM 8.2

Patient history: Mrs Jones gets severe asthma, particularly in the summer when the pollen count is high. She has just been admitted to the ward with an acute asthma attack.

Problem: Mrs Jones is experiencing difficulty in breathing due to acute severe asthma.

Goal: Mrs Jones respiratory status will return to her normal measurements.

Interventions

Mrs Jones requires all the care described for Mr Brown. However, because the cause of her respiratory distress is known it is possible to be more specific about certain aspects of her care. These are listed below, and described above in more detail, in Mr Brown's care plan. The interval between observations has not been given since the degree of her respiratory distress is not known.

● Observe and record Mrs Jones' respiratory rate, depth and rhythm every *x* hours.
● Observe for evidence of cyanosis.
● Record Mrs Jones' pulse oximetry every *x* hours.

- Record Mrs Jones' peak expiratory flow rate every x hours.
- Record Mrs Jones' blood pressure, pulse and temperature every x hours.
- Position Mrs Jones in an upright position, well supported with pillows.
- Explain all procedures and the plan of care to Mrs Jones.
- Administer oxygen as prescribed.
- Obtain sputum specimen.

Intervention: assist Mrs Jones in meeting the activities of daily living

Mrs Jones will require assistance in meeting all of her activities of daily living due to her breathlessness.

Intervention: administer nebulizers as prescribed

A nebulizer is a device that turns liquid medication into a fine mist containing particles small enough to reach deep into the bronchial tree. Nebulizers use compressed gas to change a liquid drug into a vapour, so delivering drugs into the lungs in a mist of particles small enough to reach the bronchioles and sometimes the alveoli (Muers and Corris 1997).

Nebulizers are used in preference to inhalers for adults:

- when large drug doses are needed
- when it is not possible for patients to control and coordinate their breathing to make the use of inhalers possible (e.g. in acute severe asthma or an exacerbation of COPD)
- when inhalers have been found to be ineffective in managing the patient's chronic lung disease
- when preparations such as antibiotics and lignocaine are required, since such preparations are unavailable as inhalers.

Bronchodilators, steroids, antibiotics, rhDNase, pentamadine, lignocaine and 0.9% sodium chloride are available for nebulization. Water should not be nebulized since it may cause bronchoconstriction (Muers and Corris 1997).

Nebulizers with masks are better for acutely ill patients who may find holding the nebulizer tiring.

Nebulizers with mouthpieces should be used:

- if patients find masks claustrophobic
- if steroids are being used, to prevent deposition on the face
- for nebulized antibiotics, so that a filter can be used to prevent exhalation of antibiotic into the air
- with certain anticholinergic drugs, since they may exacerbate glaucoma.

The mouth should be rinsed out after nebulizing steroids and antibiotics to prevent the development of oral thrush (Muers and Corris 1997).

ALERT!

Patients with acute severe asthma should have their nebulizers administered via oxygen or they will become hypoxic. Air should be used for all other lung diseases unless oxygen is prescribed. If necessary, low-flow oxygen can be administered via nasal cannulae to patients while a drug is nebulized with air. This is because it requires a high flow of oxygen to nebulize a drug (6–8 litres/minute) and if the patient has chronic respiratory disease he will require only a low level of oxygen to stimulate his respiration.

Intervention: to administer Mrs Jones's nebulizer

Equipment

- Appropriate gas source.
- Nebulizer and face mask/mouthpiece.
- Gas supply tubing.
- Nebulizer solution (at room temperature to prevent bronchospasm).
- Prescription chart.

Procedure

- Explain the procedure to Mrs Jones to reduce anxiety and gain consent.
- Wash hands.
- Prepare equipment.
- Assist Mrs Jones to sit upright, to allow for maximum lung expansion.
- Prepare the nebulizer solution, adhering to the guidelines set out in Chapter 6 and check Mrs Jones's identity.
- Unscrew the base of the nebulizer, add the solution to the chamber and screw the nebulizer together again.
- Attach a face mask to the nebulizer, and if necessary attach tubing to the nebulizer and attach this to the air or oxygen cylinder (depending upon prescription).
- Advise Mrs Jones that she will need to remain sitting upright, and should take normal steady breaths (tidal breathing) throughout the treatment. She should also be instructed not to talk during the nebulization and to keep the nebulizer upright.
- Set the flow meter to 6–8 litres/minute if a cylinder or piped gas is being used (Muers and Corris 1997); otherwise switch the compressor to *On* if a portable electric/battery compressor is being used.
- Assist Mrs Jones to place the mask over her nose and mouth and secure it by placing the elastic straps over the ears and back of head.
- Advise Mrs Jones to breathe normally and remain sitting upright throughout the duration of the treatment – approximately 10 minutes.
- Provide Mrs Jones with a sputum pot, tissues and mouthwash, as she is likely to need to expectorate during and after administration of the nebulizer. If antibiotics or steroids have been nebulized the patient's mouth must be washed out to prevent the development of oral candida.
- Document the therapy, any complications and the response to treatment.

Intervention: refer patient to Clinical Nurse Specialist in Respiratory Care

It is advisable to refer poorly controlled asthmatic patients to the relevant Clinical Nurse Specialist to review their asthma management.

Evaluation

Has Mrs Jones experienced relief in response to the interventions? Have her vital signs changed towards her normal parameters?

NURSING PROBLEM 8.3

Problem: Mrs Jones cannot use her inhaler correctly.
Goal: Mrs Jones will be able to demonstrate correct inhaler technique.

Intervention: using inhalers

Inhalers allow drugs to be administered directly to the lungs – thus allowing smaller doses to be used and reducing systemic side effects. An inhaler is a device consisting of a reservoir of drug, either in aerosol or powder form, and a mouthpiece through which the drug is inhaled. Devices are either activated through inspiration (breath-activated) or by manual action.

The range of drugs available and the devices for the delivery of such drugs is vast and continually developing. Drugs found in inhalers include the following.

Short-acting bronchodilators

These are also known as 'relievers'. Examples include Salbutamol and Ipratropium Bromide. These drugs have varying speeds of onset of effect. For example, Salbutamol may have an effect within 5 minutes yet Ipratropium Bromide may take 20 minutes before an effect is felt. Inhalers in this group are usually coloured blue or grey.

Long-acting bronchodilators

Salmeterol is an example of this group. These drugs have long-lasting actions (e.g. a 12-hour effect) but take longer to act initially. These drugs are therefore prescribed for regular administration, such as twice daily, rather than on an 'as required' basis. These inhalers are usually green in colour.

TIP! **For patients with persistent breathlessness, bronchodilators should be used before activity or to relieve the effort of eating.**

Inhaled steroids

These are also known as 'preventers'. These drugs have an anti-inflammatory effect. They have a slow onset of action and patients may feel no effect for several days after commencing treatment. Inhaled steroids should be taken regularly every day, even when the patient feels well, to prevent an increase in inflammatory changes in the bronchioles. These inhalers are brown/red/orange/pink in colour. The mouth should be rinsed out after inhaling steroids, to prevent the development of oral thrush.

To ensure that the maximum amount of drug is deposited in the lungs, it is imperative that an appropriate device is chosen and that the patient's technique is adequate. Many metered dose inhalers (MDIs) require considerable strength on the index finger and thumb to activate the aerosol release: finger strength, manual dexterity and coordination therefore need to be assessed. In addition, the patient's memory needs to be assessed, so that if required a simpler inhaler can be prescribed or a carer can help to give it.

Inhaler technique

Before teaching a patient it is advisable to assess his or her knowledge of the subject. This can prevent unnecessary repetition and can also identify areas of misunderstanding. In this instance you could ask Mrs Jones to tell you what she knows about her inhaler and to demonstrate how she thinks it should be used.

Everybody learns in a different way, and it is important to assess how Mrs Jones learns best. Mrs Jones may find that it is useful to learn inhaler technique by having the procedure broken into easy stages and repeating these until the final stage is learnt and the whole procedure accomplished. However, some patients feel more comfortable with written guidance, private practice and finally performance in front of a health care professional. Other patients may have problems with understanding English and others may be unable to read. Ask Mrs Jones how she learns a practical skill before you start.

Using the above information, a teaching session will need to be devised to facilitate Mrs Jones in learning to use her inhaler. In certain

Trusts a Clinical Nurse Specialist in Respiratory Care will deliver the teaching session but this varies from Trust to Trust. Mrs Jones will first need to learn about the type of inhaler she has.

The following details give the procedure for a variety of different inhalers. It is good practice to teach a patient using placebo devices. These are widely available from manufacturers, pharmacy departments and specialist nurses.

TIP! When a patient needs to take more than one inhaled drug at the same time it is usual for the short-acting bronchodilator to be administered first so that the other drugs can penetrate the lungs more efficiently.

Pressurized/aerosol metered dose inhalers (MDIs)

MDIs (Figure 8.4) are used very widely; however, many patients find it very difficult to coordinate inhalation and activation so certain inhaler devices have short spacing attachments to assist with this. For people with weak fingers or arthritis, a Haleraid hand grip may be applied to allow the inhaler to be activated by a squeezing action rather than a pressing action.

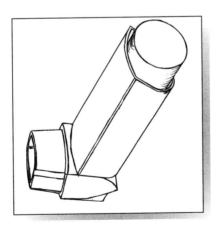

Figure 8.4
Metered dose inhaler.

Procedure for administration of MDI

- Sit or stand upright.
- Remove cap, shake inhaler.

- Breathe out gently. Place lips around mouthpiece.
- Inhale slowly and deeply through the mouth, at the same time activating the aerosol once only.
- Remove the inhaler from mouth and keep mouth closed.
- Hold the breath for 10 seconds or as long as possible.
- Repeat the procedure as required, waiting approximately 30 seconds between each activation.

Breath-actuated MDIs

These inhalers (e.g. Autohalers and Easi-breathe) are activated by the patient's inspiration. These devices can help overcome coordination problems (Figure 8.5).

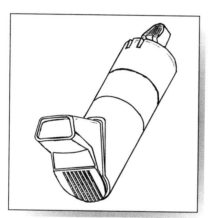

Figure 8.5.1
Autohaler.

Figure 8.5.2
Easi-breathe
device

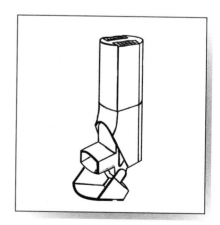

Figure 8.5.1–2 Breath-activated metered dose inhalers.

Procedure for use of the Autohaler device

- Sit or stand upright.
- Remove cap, shake inhaler.
- Breathe out gently. Place lips around mouthpiece.
- Inhale slowly and deeply through the mouth. *Do not* stop breathing when the inhaler 'clicks' – continue to take a very deep breath.
- Remove the inhaler from mouth and keep mouth closed.
- Hold the breath for 10 seconds or as long as possible.
- Repeat the procedure as required, waiting approximately 30 seconds between each activation.

NB: the lever must be pushed up (*On*) before each dose, and pushed down again (*Off*) afterwards, otherwise it will not operate.

Procedure for use of the Easi-breathe device

- Sit or stand upright.
- Hold the inhaler upright. Open cap.
- Breathe out gently. Place lips around mouthpiece.
- Inhale slowly and deeply through the mouth. *Do not* stop breathing when the inhaler 'puffs' – continue to take a very deep breath.
- Remove the inhaler from mouth and keep mouth closed.
- Hold the breath for 10 seconds or as long as possible.
- After use, hold the inhaler upright and immediately close the cap.
- Repeat the procedure as required, waiting approximately 30 seconds between each actuation.

Dry powder devices

These inhalers are triggered by a deliberate inhalation from the device. Such devices include Spinhalers, Rotahalers, Aerohalers, Aerolizers, Diskhalers, Accuhalers and Turbohalers (Figure 8.6).

All dry powder devices are loaded and prepared differently. It is advisable to consult the manufacturer's instructions for this information since it frequently changes. However, correct dry powder inhaler technique follows these general principles.

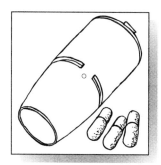

Figure 8.6.1
Spinhaler.

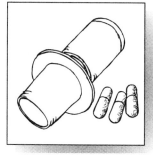

Figure 8.6.2
Rotahaler

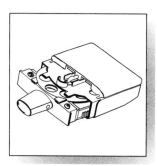

Figure 8.6.3
Aerohaler.

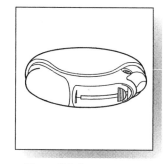

Figure 8.6.4
Accuhaler.

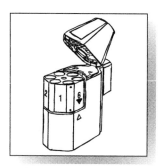

Figure 8.6.5
Diskhaler

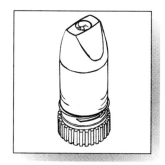

Figure 8.6.6
Turbohaler

Figure 8.6.1–6 Examples of dry powder devices.

- Load the inhaler as instructed by the manufacturer.
- Sit or stand upright.
- Breathe out gently and tilt the head back. Place lips around the mouthpiece.

- Inhale quickly and deeply through the mouth.
- Remove the inhaler from mouth and keep mouth closed.
- Hold the breath for 10 seconds or as long as possible.

Spacer devices

If a patient uses a spacer device in hospital it should be named so that others do not use it – so reducing the risk of cross-infection. Spacer devices offer the following advantages:

- There is no need to coordinate actuation of the canister with inhalation.
- There is no cold impact of cold aerosol particles on the back of the throat, which may make some people gag or cough.
- Larger drug particles, which would otherwise be deposited in the mouth and throat, are deposited in the chamber, reducing the possibility of oral candida from oral steroids.

Procedure for use of spacer devices

- Ensure that the spacer and inhaler are compatible. Each make varies and they are not interchangeable.
- Place the two halves of the spacer together.
- Remove the cap and shake the inhaler. Place mouthpiece of inhaler into port of spacer (Figure 8.7).

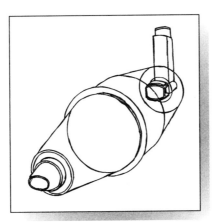

Figure 8.7
Volumatic
spacer device.

- Sit upright.
- Breathe out gently. Place lips around spacer mouthpiece.

- Hold spacer level and place one actuation into the spacer.
- Inhale slowly and deeply. If a deep inhalation is not possible the patient should breathe in deeply several times, exhaling into the canister.
- Remove the inhaler from mouth and keep mouth closed.
- Hold the breath for 10 seconds or as long as possible.
- Repeat the procedure as required, waiting approximately 30 seconds between each actuation.

Care of the spacer

The spacer should be washed each week in warm soapy water and left to dry. It is important that the inside is not wiped dry as this may damage the anti-static coating.

FIRST AID TIP!

If an individual is too breathless to use an MDI correctly and no medical aid is available, a polystyrene cup may be used as a spacer device: insert the mouthpiece of the inhaler through the bottom of a cup; place the cup, with the attached inhaler, over the individual's nose and mouth; activate the device; and encourage the casualty to breathe deeply through their nose and mouth. Seek emergency assistance.

Evaluation

In order to evaluate whether the goal has been met the following questions could be used when checking Mrs Jones's inhaler technique:

- Is Mrs Jones sitting upright?
- Has the device been prepared correctly? (For example, if using an MDI, was this shaken?)
- Has Mrs Jones taken single actuations only, i.e. not 'multi-puffing'? It is important that patients only take one puff at a time, since taking multiple inhalations at one time is ineffective and can stimulate a cough reflex.
- Has Mrs Jones inhaled sufficiently?
- Has the full dose been delivered (e.g. did any mist escape)?
- Was the breath held for at least 10 seconds?

NURSING PROBLEM 8.4

Patient history: Mr Barrett is an elderly gentleman with a chest infection, but is too weak and tired to cough and expectorate. When listening to his breathing he has a 'rattly' chest, which he and his relatives find distressing.

Problem: Mr Barrett is too weak to clear his airway effectively.

Goal: Mr Barrett's airway will remain patent.

Intervention: oropharyngeal suction

This care plan assumes that Mr Barrett is conscious. However, if he were unconscious he should be nursed on his side (to prevent his tongue blocking the airway and to facilitate the drainage of secretions) and an artificial airway may be required.

Oral or nasopharyngeal suctioning may be used. Oral suction is used for:

- unconscious or semi-conscious patients, e.g. post-operative recovery patients who are vomiting and do not have a gag reflex to prevent them from inhaling vomit or secretions
- patients who have had oral surgery or trauma resulting in blood and mucous secretions which need to be removed
- patients who are too weak to expectorate sputum from the pharynx.

Oral and nasopharyngeal suction are not the same as tracheal suction as they do not completely occlude a patient's airway. As suctioning by these routes does not enter a sterile area the procedure is clean, rather than aseptic. However, the Yankuer (oral) sucker should be used for one patient only and changed daily. It can be a very distressing procedure for the patient and should not be undertaken for prolonged periods. It may be used in conjunction with a Guedel airway if the airway needs to be maintained.

Equipment for oral suctioning

- Suction machine/piped suction.
- Suction tubing and oral suction catheter (e.g. Yankuer sucker).
- Sterile distilled water.
- Face mask.
- Eye shield.
- Towel or absorbent pad to protect patient's clothes and bed linen.
- Gloves.

Procedure for oral suctioning

- Explain procedure to Mr Barrett. (Even if the patient is unconscious explanations should be given, since many unconscious individuals are able to hear.)
- Wash hands.
- Prepare equipment.
- Attach suction tubing to suction machine and attach oral sucker to suction tubing, ensuring a tight fit.

TIP! You should regularly check that the suction machine is working and ready for use by plugging it in, switching it on and kinking the suction tubing. This should cause the pressure dial to rise. Ensure that clean suction tubing is changed between patients, and that a Yankuer (oral) sucker and flexible catheters are easily accessible to the machine.

- Position Mr Barrett in a semi-recumbent position with head turned towards you. If he is unconscious he should be nursed in a semi-prone position, facing you.
- Place a towel or pad under Mr Barrett's chin.
- Switch the suction machine on and set suction level. Oral or nasopharyngeal suction should be gentle so that the mucous membrane, teeth, or gums are not damaged. Ideal suction levels for oral suction have little supporting evidence but experience suggests that 20 kilopascals (kPa) or 120 mmHg for wall suction units is the maximum pressure.

- Put on gloves, eye shield and mask.
- Ask Mr Barrett to open his mouth and assist him if necessary.
- Insert the Yankuer sucker into the mouth along one side and guide it along the inside of the cheek towards the oropharynx without applying suction. Suction is prevented by either kinking the suction catheter or leaving the hole in the Yankuer sucker open.
- Apply suction by either unkinking the tubing or occluding the hole in the Yankuer sucker, and remove secretions and debris from mouth as required. Do not force the sucker between the teeth or touch the posterior pharyngeal wall of the soft palate as it can make the patient gag or vomit.
- Release suction and remove oral sucker from Mr Barrett's mouth. Oral suction should not be for prolonged periods as it can be very distressing to the patient.

TIP! **Hold your breath while you suction because when you feel the need to breathe again that will indicate that the episode of suctioning is long enough.**

- Clean the sucker and tubing by suctioning through sterile water until all debris has been cleared.
- If further suctioning is required allow Mr Barrett to rest for at least 30 seconds and repeat above procedure. If he is able, ask him to deep breathe and/or cough between suctions so that secretions can rise to the upper airway.
- Wash hands.
- Document the quantity, colour, consistency and odour of secretions and the patient's response to the procedure.

Intervention: nasopharyngeal suctioning

Nasopharyngeal suction is indicated when the oral sucker cannot pass to the back of the pharynx. This may be due to teeth clenching, dental or oral surgery or trauma, or if the patient cannot tolerate the Yankuer sucker at the back of the pharynx. It is particularly useful for patients with a lot of secretions at the back of the throat but who cannot cough or expectorate. It may be used in conjunction with a nasopharyngeal airway, which is tolerated quite well by semi-conscious patients.

Equipment

- Suction machine/piped suction.
- Suction tubing and sterile catheter (12–16 Fr).
- Gloves.
- Sterile distilled water.
- Face mask.
- Towel or absorbent pad to protect patient's clothes and bed linen.

Procedure

- Explain procedure to Mr Barrett. (Even if Mr Barrett is unconscious, explanations should be given, since many unconscious individuals are able to hear.)
- Wash hands.
- Prepare equipment.
- Attach suction tubing to suction machine and attach oral sucker to suction tubing, ensuring a tight fit. Check that the suction machine and equipment are working.
- Position Mr Barrett in a semi-recumbent position with head turned towards you. If he is unconscious he should be nursed semi-prone, facing you.
- Place a towel or pad under Mr Barrett's chin.
- Switch the suction machine on and set suction level for up to 20 kPa or 120 mmHg for wall suction units (see 'Oral suction'). It is important that excessive suction is not used since this may cause damage to the mucosa.
- Put on gloves, eye shield and mask.
- Attach a sterile catheter to the suction tubing and approximate the distance between the patient's ear lobe and tip of the nose, marking this point with gloved thumb and forefinger. This ensures that the catheter length inserted will remain in pharyngeal area and not enter the trachea.
- Moisten the catheter tip with sterile water and apply suction to

sterile water. This will lubricate the tip to ease insertion and ensures that the equipment is working.

- Without applying suction (see above) insert the catheter into one nostril. Guide it along the floor of the nasal cavity. If there is any obstruction, remove catheter. Apply suction and gently rotate the catheter as you withdraw it to gather secretions on removal.

- The procedure should take no longer than 15 seconds to prevent damage to the patient due to oxygen insufficiency. Observe Mr Barrett's colour and facial expression to detect signs of respiratory distress. If the procedure stimulates coughing the catheter has entered too far into the respiratory passages and should be withdrawn.

TIP! Removal of secretions from the nasopharyngeal route should not interfere with the patient's oxygen levels if done for short periods of 10–15 seconds only. It should improve the patient's comfort and breathing ability as it is an effective method of clearing the airway.

- Use the catheter once and then discard by wrapping it around your gloved hand and taking off the glove with the catheter inside.
- Clean the suction tubing by suctioning through sterile water until all debris has been cleared.
- Allow Mr Barrett to rest for at least 30 seconds before repeating the procedure. There should be an audible improvement in his breathing if suction is effective.
- Wash hands.
- Document the quantity, colour, consistency and odour of secretions and the patient's response to the procedure.

ALERT!

The older adult with cardiac or pulmonary disease may be able to tolerate only 10-second periods of suctioning since they are at greater risk of developing cardiac arrhythmia as a result of hypoxia (Perry and Potter 1998).

Intervention: refer to chest physiotherapist

Chest physiotherapy will facilitate the removal of secretions. The physiotherapist will also be able to help and teach Mr Barrett to cough effectively and assist in positioning Mr Barrett to promote postural drainage.

Evaluation

Evaluation of the care given to Mr Barrett will focus upon whether his airway remains free of secretions. If Mr Barrett's level of consciousness alters, the plan of care will need to be reviewed accordingly.

Further reading

Abley C (1997) Teaching elderly patients how to use inhalers: a study to evaluate an education programme on inhaler technique for elderly patients. Journal of Advanced Nursing 25(4): 699–708.

Bell C (1995) Is this what the doctor ordered? Accuracy of oxygen therapy prescribed and delivered in hospital. Professional Nurse 10(5): 297–300.

Cowan T (1996) Nebulisers for use in the community. Professional Nurse 12(3): 215–20.

Dodd M (1996) Nebuliser therapy: what nurses and patients need to know. Nursing Standard 10(31): 39–42.

Fell H, Boehm M (1998) Easing the discomfort of oxygen therapy. Nursing Times 94(38): 56–58.

Finkelstein L (1996) Sputum testing for TB: getting good specimens. American Journal of Nursing 96(2): 14.

Grap MJ (1998) Protocols for practice: applying research at the bedside – pulse oximetry. Critical Care Nurse 18(1): 94–99.

Hall J (1996) Evaluating asthma patient inhaler technique. Professional Nurse 11(11): 725–29.

Jain P, Kavuru MS, Emerman CL, Ahmad M (1998) Utility of peak expiratory flow monitoring. Chest: The Cardiopulmonary Journal 114(3): 861–76.

Manolio TA, Weinmann GG, Buist AS, Furberg CD, Pinsky JL, Hurd SH (1997) Pulmonary function testing in population-based studies. American Journal of Respiratory and Critical Care Medicine 156(3, Pt. 1): 1004–10.

Mathews PJ (1997) Using a peak flow meter: monitoring the air waves. Nursing 27(6): 57–59.

McConnell EA (1999) Clinical do's and don't's: performing pulse oximetry. Nursing 29(11): 17.

Muers M, Corris P (1997) Current best practice for nebuliser treatment. Thorax: the Journal of the British Thoracic Society 52(Supp. 2).

O'Callaghan C, Barry P (1997) Spacer devices in the treatment of asthma. British Medical Journal 314(7087): 1061–62.

Owen A (1998) Respiratory assessment revisited. Nursing 28(4): 48–49.

Talbot L, Curtis L (1996) The challenges of assessing skin indicators in people of color. Home Healthcare Nurse 14(3): 167–73.

Wilson J, Arnold C, Connor R, Cusson R (1996) Evaluation of oxygen delivery with the use of nasopharyngeal catheters and nasal cannulas. Neonatal Network: Journal of Neonatal Nursing 15(4): 15–22.

CHAPTER 9

Assisting patients to meet their nutritional needs

Clare Bennett

Aims and learning outcomes

This chapter discusses the effect of malnutrition upon an individual's health and how it can be prevented or corrected. By the end of the chapter you should be able to:

● define malnutrition
● discuss the incidence and impact of malnutrition in the community and hospital settings
● feed a patient via the oral route safely
● describe indications and contraindications for nasogastric tube feeding, the procedure required for tube insertion, and patient care after nasogastric tube insertion
● describe indications and contraindications for percutaneous endoscopic gastrostomy (PEG) feeding, and patient care pre- and post-insertion.

Patient assessment

Malnutrition occurs when there is an imbalance between what a person eats and what is needed physiologically. Evidence suggests that up to 10 per cent of chronically sick individuals in the community are malnourished (Edington et al. 1996), and in hospital up to 60 per cent of patients in certain wards do not consume adequate protein or calories (Bond 1997). Poor nourishment can result in various problems (Clay 2001; Ward and Rollins 1999):

- muscle atrophy
- increased risk of pressure sore development
- delayed healing
- depressed immunity
- decreased muscle strength
- increased liability to heart failure
- depression and apathy
- social isolation.

Thus, malnutrition has significant emotional, physical and economic consequences for the individual. Additionally, it presents increased costs for the health services, since it prolongs hospital admissions and requires extended treatment.

A patient's nutritional status should be assessed whether he is admitted to hospital or community care so that any indication of malnourishment can be detected early (Ward and Rollins 1999). Aspects of nutritional assessment are discussed in Chapter 1.

After assessment, a plan of care can be devised in partnership with the patient, his family/significant others, the dietician and medical colleagues to ensure that the patient's nutritional needs are met. This includes an adequate intake of proteins, fats, carbohydrates, vitamins, minerals and trace elements.

Inability to feed oneself can be due to a variety of reasons, including physical and psychological difficulties with eating. These may include:

- hemiparesis
- poor manual dexterity
- visual impairment
- swallowing problems
- lethargy
- environmental problems
- poor or lost appetite.

Although a loss of appetite will not physically prevent the patient from feeding himself it may present a significant psychological barrier. A thorough nutritional assessment may identify a specific cause and help to plan appropriate interventions.

Patients generally prefer to maintain their independence and feed themselves where possible, and this should be encouraged. Support for patients who need help to eat should be aimed at maintaining their dignity, particularly at meal times, and enabling them to regain independence. There are some suggestions here to help you provide a pleasant environment in which to eat and provide assistance for patients who cannot feed themselves. For all patients, it is essential that their appetite and intake are monitored to ensure that they are receiving an adequate nutritional intake (RCN 1996).

NURSING PROBLEM 9.1

Patient history: Mr Holmes is a 76-year-old man who has been admitted to your ward for investigations of recent weight loss and anaemia. He was widowed 12 months ago and was managing at home quite well until a bad bout of flu a month ago. He is now lethargic, disorientated and has no interest in eating.

Problem: Mr Holmes is unable to feed himself.

Goal: Mr Holmes will receive a balanced diet, totalling a calorific intake of x calories in 24 hours. (A specific time frame and measurement are not included in this example goal, as they depend on an individual's needs.)

Intervention: assisting with nutritional needs

The environment

In both the hospital and community settings environmental issues can significantly affect an individual's nutritional intake and ability or desire to feed himself. The following interventions may help Mr Holmes if this is contributing to his problem:

- Particular food preferences and needs should be identified and met (e.g. texture, diabetic diet, vegetarian diet).
- Mr Holmes should be positioned upright if possible so that he can see and easily reach his food and drinks.
- If required, appropriate use of dentures should be made. Check that these fit correctly, and arrange for dental assessment if neces-

sary. Some patients avoid going to the dentist and then cannot eat because of tooth decay and oral discomfort.

- Mr Holmes should be given a choice as to whether he wishes to eat in privacy or with others. Meals are a social occasion and people may eat more in company. The exception to this is if other people's eating habits are a distraction for Mr Holmes.
- The eating environment should be free of reminders of treatments and unpleasant odours.
- Mouth care prior to food and drink may be required to remove any unpleasant tastes from the mouth associated with treatments or infection.
- Mr Holmes should be offered the opportunity to visit the toilet and wash his hands prior to meal times.

Lethargy

- Frequently offer small quantities of well-presented food.
- Nutritional supplements, designed to provide additional protein, energy and nutrients in powder, liquid or as dessert, may help. These can be divided up and given at suitable moments during the day to boost energy intake. These may need to be prescribed and advice should be sought from the dietician regarding the most appropriate supplement for Mr Holmes's specific needs. Food fortification may also be required (see 'Poor appetite', page 218).
- Mr Holmes may get tired and need help to complete his meal. The nurse should watch for this and not assume that if food is left on a plate the patient does not want any more; he may simply be too exhausted to feed himself further.

Hemiparesis

- A plate guard and non-slip mat may help if Mr Holmes is only able to use one hand to eat. Using a feeding beaker may help if he has a one-sided weakness to the mouth.
- Nutritional supplements and food fortification may be required if Mr Holmes finds feeding particularly tiring.

Poor manual dexterity

- The occupational therapy department may be able to provide special equipment such as cutlery with enlarged handles to assist Mr Holmes.

- The nurse should give assistance with opening awkward packaging such as yoghurt tops and sandwich containers.
- It may be useful to cut up Mr Holmes's food for him. This should be done sensitively so that Mr Holmes does not feel he has regressed to childhood.

Visual impairment

- A non-slip mat and plate guard may be useful depending upon the severity of Mr Holmes's impairment.
- Orientate Mr Holmes to where things are on the plate. Clock face positions may be useful, e.g. 'The salad is at five o'clock, the chicken is at twelve o'clock', etc.

Poor appetite

- If Mr Holmes has a reduced appetite it is essential that every mouthful is full of calories and nutrients. Ledger (2000) suggests that a fortified diet which consists largely of high calorie and protein food allows a patient to increase his nutritional intake without increasing the volume of food consumed. Copeman (1999) suggests methods of food fortification such as the addition of cream, milk, butter, extra meat or grated cheese to dishes, and making soups, drinks, sauces and puddings with full-fat milk.
- Offer small quantities of food often.
- Snacks of biscuits, cakes, cheese and biscuits, yoghurts, and trifles may enhance nutritional intake.
- Nutritional supplements may be of use.
- The environmental issues should be considered.
- Offer sherry before meals as an appetizer, or a glass of Guinness or stout with the main meal to stimulate the appetite.

Swallowing problems (dysphagia)

- If Mr Holmes has dysphagia it is important to ensure his safety during feeding. A speech and language therapist should assess the degree of dysphagia and the dietician should recommend an appropriate diet.
- Puréed and soft foods such as soft minced meat, flaked fish, soft vegetables, mashed potatoes, milk puddings, scrambled eggs, and yoghurts may be both safe and acceptable to Mr Holmes. Bond

(1997) stresses that the presentation of food is extremely important; she suggests the use of thickening agents to make puréed
food look like it did before it was put into the food processor.

- Thickening agents added to drinks may help swallowing depending upon the speech and language therapist's assessment.
- Observe Mr Holmes for choking when commencing a pureeed or
  soft diet.

Evaluation

Mr Holmes may respond to some of these measures to improve his food
intake. Take note of the interventions that help him and persist with
them until his needs change.

Intervention: feeding patients

If Mr Holmes is unable to feed himself he should be helped to eat. The
following guidelines will help you to perform this role whilst maintaining the patient's dignity:

- Establish whether there are any dietary restrictions, or contraindi-
  cations to oral feeding.
- Consider environmental issues.
- Wash and dry hands and put on an appropriately coloured apron.
- Obtain the items that Mr Holmes would like to drink and/or eat,
  appropriate cutlery and a napkin.
- Present the meal as attractively as possible, place the meal on a
  table in front of Mr Holmes and place a seat to one side for yourself.
- Protect Mr Holmes's clothes with the napkin.
- Sit down and start to feed Mr Holmes. Allow him to direct the
  order in which he wishes to eat the food. Allow time for him to
  empty his mouth completely between each spoonful, aiming to
  match the speed of feeding to his readiness. Ask Mr Holmes
  whether the speed at which you are feeding him is acceptable. Try
  to engage in conversation about everyday topics to create a more
  relaxed atmosphere, but avoid asking questions when Mr Holmes
  is eating.
- Remove any spillages on the chin, face and neck with a napkin.
- If Mr Holmes likes to drink during his meal ensure you offer him
  fluids at appropriate intervals.

- When Mr Holmes has eaten as much as he can help him to clean his mouth if he so wishes.
- Remove any unwanted food and crockery, wipe up any spillages, and arrange Mr Holmes's water and personal items so that they are within reach.
- Remove apron, wash hands, document intake on fluid balance chart and/or care plan. Report any problems such as choking, vomiting or refusal to a senior colleague.

TIP! **Family members often like to help their relatives eat. If this is acceptable to the patient a relative may be encouraged to assist at meal times. This may bring comfort to both the patient and the carer.**

Evaluation

Has Mr Holmes increased his food intake? Is his appetite improving? Is he increasingly independent at meal times? Is Mr Holmes receiving an adequate balanced diet for his needs? If eating aids are being used, were they suitable and did he use them?

Monitoring these factors will indicate whether the care plan is effective.

Enteral feeding by nasogastric tube

A nasogastric (NG) tube can be used either for feeding (via a fine-bore tube) or for gastric drainage (via a Ryles tube). The focus of this care will be on feeding via a nasogastric tube. A nasogastric tube is placed directly into the stomach via the nose.

Nasogastric tube feeding may be required for:

- short-term nutritional support
- conditions where patients are unable to meet their nutritional needs by mouth although they have a functioning gastro-intestinal tract: e.g. fractured jaw; loss of swallowing reflex; inflammation of the mouth or throat, for example, following radiotherapy
- supplementing oral intake: e.g. when patients have a depressed appetite; carcinomas; inflammatory illnesses such as Crohn's disease; chronic system failure such as renal failure

● metabolic abnormalities
● hypercatabolic states: e.g. sepsis; burns; major trauma, including surgery
● psychological problems causing loss of appetite.

Contraindications to NG feeding include:

● intestinal obstruction
● paralytic ileus
● diffuse peritonitis
● intractable vomiting
● severe diarrhoea
● severe malabsorption
● short bowel syndrome
● certain cases of severe pancreatitis, high output gastro-intestinal fistulae and gastro-intestinal ischaemia, although enteral nutrition may sometimes still be feasible
● basal skull fractures
● when prolonged feeding is required (longer than 2–4 weeks).

Choosing the appropriate tube

Ryles tubes should not be sited specifically for enteral feeding; they should only be sited if monitoring of gastric absorption is required. Ryles tubes are available in sizes 9–22 FG. They are made of PVC and are therefore quite rigid. Their large size and rigidity are associated with a number of complications: discomfort; ulceration of oesophageal and nasal tissue; difficulties in swallowing solid food; gastro-oesophageal reflux; rhinitis; pharyngitis; oesophagitis; oesophageal erosion and stricture; upper GI bleeding; and pneumothorax (Kennedy 1997).

Fine-bore tubes are much smaller. They are available in sizes 6–9 FG and are made of polyurethane which is a soft material. Patients generally find these tubes much more comfortable than Ryles tubes and are usually unaware of the tube within a few hours following insertion, which allows them to eat and drink normally. These tubes are associated with fewer complications than the Ryles tube. However, they are unsuitable for aspirating large amounts from the stomach. Fine-bore tubes can be left in situ for between one and several weeks depending upon their construction materials. Standard feeds can be administered via a 6 Fr tube; more viscous feeds such as those containing fibre should be delivered via an 8 Fr tube to prevent tube occlusion (Rollins 1997).

NURSING PROBLEM 9.2

Patient history: Mr Palmer is 66, and has been diagnosed with a stroke affecting his left cerebral hemisphere that has affected his speech and swallowing mechanisms and resulted in a right hemiparesis (paralysis of the right side).

Problem: Mr Palmer cannot eat enough orally to meet his nutritional needs due to an impaired swallowing reflex following a stroke.

Goal: Mr Palmer will receive a balanced nutritional intake, totalling a calorific intake of x calories in 24 hours via a nasogastric tube.

Intervention: inserting a nasogastric tube

Equipment

- Appropriately sized fine-bore tube.
- Receiver.
- Sterile water or 0.9% sodium chloride.
- Blue litmus paper/pH test strips.
- Clean disposable gloves.
- Glass of water and straw (if drinking is not contraindicated).
- Tissues.
- 50 ml syringe.
- Stethoscope.
- Spigot (if using Ryles tube).
- Securing tape.
- Scissors.
- Disposable apron.
- Vomit bowl.

Procedure

● A detailed explanation of the procedure should be given to Mr Palmer as many patients find nasogastric tube insertion distressing. Mr Palmer should be shown the tube and the entire procedure explained. Be aware that Mr Palmer may consider his body image to be altered and may require support to cope with this.

● Check for allergies to adhesive tape.

● Prepare equipment.

● Assist Mr Palmer to sit up comfortably with a straight body and his neck in a relaxed position (either flexed or extended).

● Decide which nostril to use – ask Mr Palmer about blockages, breaks, fractures, polyps or previous surgery to the nose. Establish if he has a preference and ask him to breathe through each nostril separately to detect any obstruction.

● Ask Mr Palmer to blow his nose.

● Wash hands.

● Put on apron and clean disposable gloves.

● Remove the tube from its packaging and stretch it to remove any shape retained from the packaging. This will aid passage of the tube and make it easier to remove the guide wire (if present) once the tube has been passed.

● Measure the length from Mr Palmer's ear lobe to the bridge of his nose, plus the distance from the bridge of the nose to the base of the sternum (xiphisternum) (Figure 9.1). Mark this length on the tube with a marker pen.

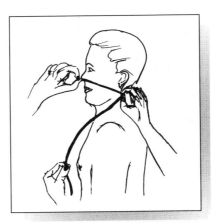

Figure 9.1
Measuring the length of an NG tube.

- Agree a signal with Mr Palmer by which he can indicate that he needs a break if necessary.
- If using a fine-bore tube follow the manufacturer's guidelines regarding tube preparation – this may include ensuring that the guide wire is firmly anchored in the tube, and flushing it with 0.9% sodium chloride or water and dipping the end of the tube in water. If using a Ryles tube, dip the end in water.
- If Mr Palmer is able to swallow safely, give him the glass of water with a straw.
- Introduce the tube into the chosen nostril and gently slide it along the floor of the nose towards the nasopharynx approximately 15 cm.
- Ask Mr Palmer to put his chin on his chest and take a sip of water and hold this in his mouth. As he swallows advance the tube 10–15 cm and stop.

ALERT!

If the patient shows signs of distress, e.g. coughing, gasping or breathlessness, remove the tube immediately as it may have entered the bronchus.

- If Mr Palmer is calm, with no signs of distress, continue to advance the tube while he sips and swallows the water, until the marked length has been reached.
- Lightly secure the tape, temporarily, ensuring it is comfortable.
- Attach the syringe to the guide wire/tube and aspirate a small amount of stomach contents. This should be yellow/green clear fluid. Drop some of the aspirate on to the blue litmus paper; since gastric contents are acidic, the aspirate should turn blue litmus paper red, rapidly and definitely.
- In some Trusts, more specific pH testing is required, using pH test paper. This will give an indication to the nearest half unit. Gastric acid has a pH < 3 (less than 3) whereas bronchial secretions have a pH > 6 (greater than 6) (Rollins 1997). The only exception to this is if a patient is receiving medication to control gastric acid. If this is the case, a chest X-ray will be required to confirm correct placement.

● If the aspirate results suggest that the tube is correctly positioned, rapidly inject 20–30 ml air into the tube (without removing the guide wire) whilst listening over the epigastrum with a stethoscope.

ALERT!

Auscultation (listening) alone is not sufficient to confirm the correct position of the tube since it is very easy to misinterpret where the air sounds are coming from. Both litmus testing and auscultation are necessary.

Recommended practice requires that an abdominal X-ray should confirm correct positioning. If there is any doubt about the position of the tube, or if it has been difficult to pass, a chest X-ray should be carried out to ensure that it is not in the lungs, before any feed is commenced (Loan et al. 1998).

● If a fine-bore tube has been used, when correct positioning has been confirmed remove the guide wire by holding the feeding tube firmly at the nose using gentle traction, and withdraw the guide wire gently. It may be necessary to instil 5 ml of water to activate the lubricant prior to applying traction, depending upon the brand of tube used.

ALERT!

Never reinsert a guide wire once it has been removed.

● Firmly secure the tube using soft tape in a position that is acceptable to Mr Palmer, for example, under his cheekbone, and loop it over the ear.
● Help Mr Palmer to assume a more comfortable position, and provide all he needs within easy reach.
● Dispose of equipment, remove gloves, wash hands.
● Record all actions in Mr Palmer's documentation.

TIP! If inserting a Ryles tube, it may slip down more easily if it is cold. Place it in the freezer compartment for an hour before insertion.

Intervention: maintaining the patency of the tube

- Flush the tube with water before and after feeding; and before, after and between the administration of medication; 6-hourly flushes are recommended if feeding continuously (Colagiovanni 2000).
- Research has not yet confirmed the quantity of water that should be used for flushing, although Burnham (2000) recommends a minimum of 20 ml.
- If the tube is not being used, it should be flushed regularly with water, although research has not identified the frequency for flushing. Common sense would suggest 6-hourly flushing although there is little supporting evidence for this.
- Polyurethane tubes are preferable to silicone tubes as they appear to block less readily (Colagiovanni 2000).
- When administering medication, dispersible preparations should be used where possible and syrups should be diluted with water. If tablets have to be crushed they should be mixed thoroughly with water prior to administration. If more than one drug is required, the tube should be flushed with water between each drug (Colagiovanni 2000; see Chapter 6).
- If 4–6-hourly aspiration is required to assess gastric absorption, tubes are more likely to become blocked. It is therefore advisable to use a wide-bore tube until gastric emptying is confirmed, and then replace it with a fine-bore tube (Colagiovanni 2000).
- If the tube blocks, water or carbonated drinks may be useful in dispersing food clots (Colagiovanni 2000). Force should not be used to introduce these substances as this may cause the tube to split (Baeyens et al. 1999).

ALERT!

When flushing the tube, the manufacturer's guidelines regarding syringe size must be adhered to, to prevent splitting of the tube. Generally syringes need to be greater than 30 ml (Rollins 1997).

Intervention: administering NG feed as prescribed

The type of feed prescribed will depend upon Mr Palmer's needs. Many different types are available including:

- whole protein mixtures which require normal digestion
- semi-elemental or elemental feeds which require minimum digestion and are readily absorbed in the upper gut
- specialist feeds for people in renal failure, or children.

Feeds are usually given continuously or overnight, although occasionally some patients may have bolus feeds at their usual meal times.

ALERT!

The position of the tube must be checked every 24 hours, and after physiotherapy, vomiting, regurgitation or violent coughing.

Equipment to administer a continuous feed

- Functioning enteral feeding tube.
- Administration set (with container if using canned feed).
- Appropriate feed prescribed by dietician.
- Sterile water.
- A clean and operational feeding pump.
- 50 ml syringe.
- Feeding regimen.

Procedure to administer a continuous feed

- Prepare equipment.
- Explain procedure to Mr Palmer.
- Wash hands.
- Confirm correct position of tube using litmus test, auscultation and X-ray as described above.
- Wash hands.
- Flush tube with a minimum of 20 ml water (Burnham 2000).
- Wash hands.

- If using feed in a can, using a non-touch technique carefully decant the feed into the bag of the administration set and hang the bag. If using a bottle feed, shake the container vigorously. Hold the bottle upright; without touching the foil seal, unscrew and remove the plastic cap. Do not puncture or attempt to remove the foil seal. Open the giving set and screw firmly onto the top of the bottle. The spike of the giving set will automatically break the foil seal. Invert and hang bottle using the integral hook.
- Prime the administration set by opening the clamp and allowing the feed to flow to the end.
- Position the administration set into the pump according to manufacturer's instructions.
- Attach administration set to feeding tube.
- Set flow rate and start the pump.
- Observe for signs of respiratory distress such as breathlessness, cyanosis, and difficulty in breathing. If these should occur stop feed immediately and inform senior colleague.
- Record feed on fluid balance chart.
- Label administration set with date and time commenced.
- Each time the feed is stopped or changed flush the tube with a minimum of 20 ml water (Burnham 2000).
- Document all actions in Mr Palmer's records.
- Leave call bell within easy reach of Mr Palmer and instruct him to alert you if he should experience any respiratory difficulty or abdominal discomfort.
- Change the administration set and bag every 24 hours.

Procedure to administer feeds by bolus

- Check position of tube as described previously.
- Attach syringe barrel without the internal piston to tube, kink the tube to prevent flow and fill with required fluid.
- Release kink and empty gradually, raising or lowering the height of the barrel to control the speed of flow.
- Refill and repeat until prescribed amount has been given.

TIP! **Patients who are fed exclusively by fluid feed may develop either constipation or diarrhoea. Observe the frequency and consistency of the patient's faeces and report abnormalities to senior staff and the dietician, as altering the constituents of the feed may relieve the problem.**

Enteral feeding: a patient's comfort needs

Mr Palmer will require a separate care plan to address his comfort needs. This would include the following interventions:

● Clean facial skin daily with mild soap and water depending on a patient's preference; dry thoroughly and apply fresh tape.
● Clean nostrils daily, removing crusts and discharge.
● Check for skin erosions on nasal mucosa, the edge of the nostrils, skin underneath the tube and behind the ears.
● Alter the position of the tube to relieve these areas on the face and ears frequently.
● Provide regular oral hygiene, especially if Mr Palmer is not able to take anything orally.

Evaluation

Has Mr Palmer received a balanced diet by NG tube? Is he able to absorb the tube feed? Has his skin remained intact?

Intervention: insertion and care of a percutaneous endoscopic gastrostomy (PEG) tube

A gastrostomy is an artificial opening through the abdominal wall into the stomach, through which a feeding tube is passed. The tube is usually inserted endoscopically and is therefore known as a percutaneous endoscopic gastrostomy.

Indications for a PEG include long-term feeding as for a nasogastric tube, or for conditions requiring enteral feeding for more than two weeks, and an inability to tolerate NG tubes (Reilly 1998; Arrowsmith 1996).

PEG tubes are contraindicated for the same conditions as NG tubes except for basal skull fractures and prolonged feeding. The British Society of Gastroenterology (1996) and Arrowsmith (1996) also note that additional contraindications are:

● patient unfit for endoscopy
● current chest infection
● ascites
● portal hypertension (with gastric varices)

- active gastric ulcer
- total gastrectomy
- uncorrected coagulopathy (blood clotting dysfunction).

Some advantages of a PEG are:

- more comfortable than an NG tube
- cosmetically more acceptable for some patients
- reduced risk of tube displacement
- reduced risk of tube blockage
- does not need regular replacement.

NURSING PROBLEM 9.3

Patient history: Mr Hamilton has had surgery for cancer of the oesophagus and will be unable to take fluid and diet by the oral route for some time until his treatment is complete. He is to have a percutaneous endoscopic gastrostomy (PEG) tube inserted for all his nutritional needs.

Problem: Mr Hamilton needs to be physically and psychologically prepared for a percutaneous endoscopic gastrostomy (PEG).

Goal: Mr Hamilton will be physically and psychologically prepared for the procedure.

Intervention: preparing a patient for a PEG

To prepare Mr Hamilton for the procedure, Arrowsmith (1996) recommends the following interventions:

- Discuss the procedure and aftercare with Mr Hamilton, allowing him adequate time to ask questions. Mr Hamilton may understand the procedure and its implications more clearly if a diagram is used. He may appreciate the opportunity to see an example of the tube beforehand, and to discuss the changes in lifestyle and altered body image that will affect him. An experienced nurse may help Mr Hamilton make some significant psychological adjustments (White 2000). Some Trusts have specialist nutrition nurses available for counselling prior to the procedure.

- Ensure that Mr Hamilton will have nil by mouth for 6 hours prior to the procedure to prevent aspiration. This should be explained clearly to Mr Hamilton so that he appreciates that the successful outcome of the procedure requires an empty stomach.
- Ensure that written consent is obtained and that details of explanations of the procedure are documented in Mr Hamilton's records.
- Ensure that Mr Hamilton's full blood count and clotting levels are recorded. It is essential that appropriate doctors are made aware of the results in case there are abnormalities to be corrected.
- Administer any prescribed sedation and prophylactic antibiotics. This ensures Mr Hamilton is comfortable and relaxed, and potential infection from flora from the gastrointestinal tract is limited.

Evaluation

Did Mr Hamilton undergo the procedure with minimal discomfort? Were all his questions answered beforehand? Has he adapted fully to the change to PEG tube?

NURSING PROBLEM 9.4

Problem: Mr Hamilton is at risk of infection and tube blockage as he has a newly formed PEG in situ.

Goal: Infection will be prevented and the patency of the PEG will be maintained.

Intervention: post-insertion care

To prevent infection following the insertion of a PEG, Arrowsmith (1996) advocates the following interventions:

- Record Mr Hamilton's temperature, pulse and blood pressure every 30 minutes for 2 hours, then hourly for 2 hours or until stable, to detect signs of hypovolaemia and/or septic shock. Continue observations every 4 hours for 5 days or until Mr Hamilton is showing no signs of post-insertion complications such as septicaemia, stoma site infection or bleeding.
- Ensure that Mr Hamilton fasts for at least 6 hours post-insertion. After this time, if bowel sounds are present and there is no abdominal pain, pyrexia or tachycardia, water is given at a rate of 85 ml/hour for the next 6 hours. If there is no nausea or abdominal distension, the feed is commenced according to the dietician's instructions. It is usual to start off slowly, then gradually increase the rate. If nausea or abdominal distension occurs, the rate should be reduced; if the symptoms are severe, it should be stopped.
- Inspect the site under the fixation device for any blood, serous fluid or signs of inflammation. If there are signs of inflammation, obtain and send a swab for microscopy, culture and sensitivity and inform medical team. If there is any leakage clean the site with 0.9% sodium chloride and apply a keyhole dressing.
- Until the site has healed (5–14 days), clean the site with sterile 0.9% sodium chloride and dress with a dry dressing. Subsequently the site can be washed daily with soap and water, using a disposable flannel which is changed daily, and thoroughly dried. A dressing is not necessary unless there is a heavy discharge.
- After 24 hours, rotate the tube daily in a complete circle to prevent adherence to the tract.
- Leave the external fixation device intact for 72 hours to minimize gastric leakage and to encourage the stomach to adhere to the abdominal wall. Four days after insertion, release the fixation plate (noting the number mark on the tube) to access the stoma site for thorough cleaning. This should then be done daily, with the plate being replaced to its original position. Fastening too tightly may restrict blood flow and lead to tissue necrosis. If fastened too far from the stoma site, the tubing will slide in and out of the stomach and provide a route for leakage of gastric contents, resulting in infection, stoma site prolapse, formation of granulating tissue at the stoma site or bleeding.

Intervention: maintaining patency of PEG tube

To maintain patency of the PEG tube, Arrowsmith (1996) recommends the following procedures:

- Clamp for the minimum time necessary, using the plastic clamp provided by the manufacturers. A metal clamp should never be used. The tube should be closed but does not need to be clamped when it is not in use.
- Flush with water before and after feeding, and before, after and between the administration of medication.
- If not in use, flush the tube regularly with water.
- When administering medication, use dispersible preparations where possible and dilute syrups with water. If tablets have to be crushed they should be mixed thoroughly with water prior to administration. If more than one drug is required the tube should be flushed with water between each drug (Colagiovanni 2000).

Evaluation

Evaluation of the care provided will focus upon whether infection was prevented and the patency of the PEG maintained.

NURSING PROBLEM 9.5

Problem: Mr Hamilton is unable to maintain an adequate nutritional status orally, as he is unable to swallow.

Goal: Mr Hamilton will receive a balanced nutritional intake, totalling a calorific intake of x calories in 24 hours via his PEG.

Intervention: administration of a PEG feed

To administer a PEG feed, the same guidelines provided for NG tube feeding may be used. However, it is not necessary to check for correct positioning of the tube.

Evaluation

Has Mr Hamilton received a balanced diet and the required number of calories? This will be measured through accurate recording of the daily nutritional intake. If the goal has not been reached, the plan of care will need to be revised accordingly.

Further reading

ACHCEW (1997) Hungry in Hospital? London: Association of Community Health Councils of England and Wales.

Arrowsmith H (1997) Malnutrition in hospital: detection and consequences. British Journal of Nursing 6(19): 1131–35.

Baker F, Smith L, Stead L, Soulsby C (1999) Inserting a nasogastric tube. Nursing Times 95(7), Insert 2p.

Bliss DZ, Lehmann S (1999) Tube feeding: administration tips. Registered Nurse 62(8): 29–32.

Buckley PM, MacFie J (1997) Enteral nutrition in critically ill patients – a review. Care of the Critically Ill 13(1): 7–10.

Carriquiry AL (1999) Assessing the prevalence of nutrient inadequacy. Public Health Nutrition 2(1): 23–33.

Cortis JD (1997) Nutrition and the hospitalized patient. British Journal of Nursing 6(12): 666–74.

Guenter P, Jones S, Ericson M (1997) Enteral nutrition therapy. Nursing Clinics of North America 32(4): 651–68.

Lord LM (1997) Enteral access devices. Nursing Clinics of North America 32(4): 685–704.

Perry L (1997) Nutrition: a hard nut to crack. An exploration of the knowledge, attitudes and activities of qualified nurses in relation to nutritional nursing care. Journal of Clinical Nursing 6(4): 315–24.

White G (1998) Nutritional supplements and tube feeds: what is available? British Journal of Nursing 7(5): 246, 248–50.

CHAPTER 10

Elimination

Clare Bennett and Barbara Workman

Aims and learning outcomes

This chapter aims to help you to develop a sensitive, problem-focused approach to the nursing care of individuals who are experiencing difficulties with elimination. By the end of the chapter you should be able to:

- perform urinalysis
- obtain the following specimens: mid-stream urine; catheter specimen of urine; faecal specimen collection; and 24-hour urine collection
- assist with toileting, using a toilet, bedpan, urinal and commode
- apply a penile sheath
- perform catheter care
- carry out fundamental aspects of stoma care
- care for the patient who is experiencing nausea and vomiting.

Elimination

Alterations in the usual pattern of elimination may be related to a wide variety of factors including:

- reduced mobility
- infection of the gut and/or urinary tract
- medication

- neurological dysfunction
- confusion
- emotional disturbances
- disease in another system resulting in dysfunction of gastrointestinal or urinary system (e.g. diarrhoea due to hyperthyroidism).

Assessment of the usual elimination habits is therefore vital in identifying the underlying problem and planning care appropriately. This should be approached delicately since elimination is a deeply intimate and personal issue for the majority of people. Privacy should always be provided and sensitivity shown in addressing the following topics:

- Prior to the onset of the presenting problem, what were the patient's usual patterns of elimination?
- When did the usual pattern change?
- Was the change associated with any concurrent illness or events?
- What are the problems now?
- Is any pain experienced on elimination?
- What do laboratory test results and other investigations suggest?
- How is the patient coping with the current problem both physically and emotionally, and what would he like the outcomes to be?

Once this information has been collected, more specific questions relating to the problem can be asked (see care plans) and care can be planned accordingly. The following care plans focus upon various aspects of elimination. Specific time frames and measurements have not been included as these would be dependent upon the patient's condition.

Terminology

There are a number of terms that are used in hospital that patients and junior staff may not be familiar with. Here are some examples.

BNO	bowels not open
BO	bowels open
defaecation	opening the bowels
emesis	vomit

frequency	the urge to pass urine/open bowels very often
haematemesis	vomiting blood
haematuria	blood in urine
HNPU	has not passed urine
melaena	dark tarry stool indicating bleeding from the GI tract
micturition	the act of passing urine
PU	passing urine
stools	faeces
straining at stool	trying hard to pass faeces
urgency	the need to pass urine/open bowels quickly, often with little warning
voiding	emptying the bladder
+	plus sign indicating amount of urine, faeces or discharge: + indicates a small amount; ++ a moderate amount; +++ a lot.

NURSING PROBLEM 10.1

Patient history: Mrs Adams developed frequency and urgency of passing urine some time ago. She is now complaining of complete loss of bladder control on occasions.

Problem: Mrs Adams has developed urinary incontinence.

Goal: To detect underlying cause within x days.

Intervention: obtain a detailed history

To promote continence it is necessary to identify the cause of incontinence. There are numerous causes of urinary incontinence including:

- urinary tract infection
- reduced manual dexterity
- depression
- restricted mobility

- urethral sphincter incompetence
- detrusor (bladder) muscle instability
- neurological impairment
- pelvic floor weakness.

A detailed history will help to identify the underlying cause. Information needs to be obtained regarding the following issues:

- What are Mrs Adams's symptoms?
- When did the problem start?
- Does Mrs Adams pass urine when she coughs, sneezes or laughs?
- Are there problems during the day or just in the morning or at night?
- Is Mrs Adams constipated?
- Is Mrs Adams's cognitive function impaired?
- Can Mrs Adams manage to dress and undress herself, i.e. is her manual dexterity impaired?
- Is mobility reduced, making it difficult for her to get to the toilet?
- Have there been any changes in Mrs Adams's living arrangements that may make the toilet difficult to get to?
- Has Mrs Adams made any changes to her oral intake of fluids?
- Does voiding cause any pain (dysuria)?
- Is there a past history of disorders of the urinary system or disorders affecting the urinary system, such as diabetes mellitus or hypertension?
- What were Mrs Adams's usual elimination habits compared to her current pattern of elimination?
- Have there been any changes in colour, odour, consistency and volume of urine?
- Does she have sudden urgency or no warning at all of the desire to pass water?
- Has Mrs Adams had a raised temperature (pyrexia)?
- What medication does Mrs Adams take (prescribed and non-prescribed)?
- What is Mrs Adams's treatment goal?

Intervention: perform urinalysis

The term 'urinalysis' refers to the testing of urine for a variety of substances. The results of the test provide immediate information concerning the patient's kidneys, urinary tract and liver as well as information concerning other systemic functions, such as metabolism and endocrine function.

Urine reagent sticks usually test for:

- specific gravity (normal range 1005–1030)
- pH (normal range 4.5–8.0)
- protein
- glucose
- ketones
- blood
- bilirubin.

The latter two are negative in normal urine.

There are also strips available to test for additional substances or sometimes just one or very few substances.

Equipment

- Reagent strips and bottle. Check that these are in date and have been stored with the top firmly closed to prevent moisture coming into contact with the reagents.
- Receiver.
- Watch with second hand.
- Pen for use in sluice.
- Results sheet/piece of paper.
- Gloves and apron.

Procedure

- Prepare equipment.
- When Mrs Adams is able, ask her to void into the receiver. Placing a bedpan liner inside the toilet seat may do this most easily. Patients may be able to void straight into a clean universal container. This is desirable since it reduces the chances of contaminating the sample.

 First voided morning urine is best for a urinalysis as it is most concentrated (Baillie and Arrowsmith 2001).

- Put on gloves and apron and take specimen to the sluice.
- Remove a reagent stick from container and replace lid. Immerse all the reagent areas in the urine and remove immediately. Tap stick against side of container to remove excess urine.
- Note position of second hand on watch.
- Hold the strip horizontally to prevent mixing of the reagent chemicals and prevent soiling of the hands with urine.
- At the stated time on the reagent bottle, compare the test areas with the corresponding chart on the bottle (Figure 10.1).
- Make a note of the results on the urinalysis results sheet or a piece of paper. The patient's notes should not be taken into the sluice.
- Discard urine and place stick and receiver in clinical waste bin.
- Remove gloves and apron.
- Wash hands.
- Document results in Mrs Adams's notes and inform her of the results and their significance. Inform senior and medical colleagues of result.

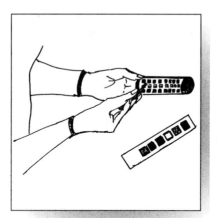

Figure 10.1
Urinalysis.

TIP! NAD means nothing abnormal detected and is a shorthand often used to record findings.

Intervention: obtain a midstream urine (MSU) specimen

MSU specimens are usually required for microscopy, culture and sensitivity (MC and S). 'Microscopy' identifies abnormal urine constituents such as blood cells, casts, pus and bacteria through the use of a microscope; 'culture' involves incubating the sample to check for the growth of organisms, and 'sensitivity' examines which treatments can be used to remove the organisms.

When obtaining an MSU specimen, the aim is to catch the middle part of the flow of urine in a single void. Since it is likely to be used for MC and S it is important that the specimen does not become contaminated with bacteria from the genital area. However, the value of cleansing the perineal/meatal area before collection of the specimen is debated in the literature. According to a meta-analysis by Brown et al. (1991), there is some doubt regarding the effectiveness of perineal/meatal cleansing. Baillie and Arrowsmith (2001) contend that such cleansing may not be necessary since the first part of the stream of urine should flush the urethra free from micro-organisms and urine should not become contaminated from the perineum if there is sufficient flow. This appears to be a sensible argument, but there is a lack of evidence available to support or refute this. It is therefore advised that you follow local policy until further evidence becomes available.

TIP! **It may be difficult to obtain an MSU specimen from Mrs Adams because of her incontinence. It may help to give her a drink, and then half an hour later take her to the toilet in the hope that she will be able to void. You may need to help her catch the specimen.**

Equipment

- Toilet or commode or bedpan.
- Sterile specimen pot.
- Laboratory request form.
- Disposable gloves.
- Apron.
- Cleansing agents as advised by local Trust policy.

Procedure

- Prepare equipment.
- Instruct or assist Mrs Adams to cleanse the perineal area as per local policy.

- Ask Mrs Adams to void and discard the initial stream of urine, then collect the middle part of the stream of urine in the sterile container, and then complete urinating in toilet/commode/bedpan. If Mrs Adams requires assistance, the nurse should wear gloves and an apron.
- Assist Mrs Adams in making herself comfortable and to wash her hands.
- Label the container clearly with Mrs Adams's name, identity number/address, date of birth, date and time collected, and examination required. Place in plastic specimen bag.
- Place specimen in refrigerator and ensure that it is transported to the laboratory promptly.
- Remove gloves and apron.
- Wash hands.
- Document collection of specimen in Mrs Adams's notes.

TIP! **The first voided morning urine is best for an MSU as it is most concentrated (Baillie and Arrowsmith 2001).**

Intervention: prepare Mrs Adams for any further investigations

Further investigations may include:

- examination of abdomen for palpable mass or bladder retention
- examination of the perineum to identify prolapse and excoriation and assess pelvic floor contraction
- rectal examination to exclude faecal impaction
- assessment of manual dexterity
- blood tests to examine blood chemistry, electrolytes, haematological profile and renal function
- tests to assess glomerular filtration rate and tubular function
- a scan of kidneys, bladder and urethra
- cystoscopy
- computerized axial tomography
- renal angiography
- urodynamic investigations.

Psychological preparation for these tests will include a full explanation of the investigation and the care required both before and after the procedure. Mrs Adams should be given written literature concerning the investigation and encouraged to ask questions. Physical preparation should reflect local protocols.

TIP! **The most recent best practice guide for continence services can be downloaded from http://www.doh.gov.uk/continence-services.htm.**

Evaluation

Has the cause of incontinence been identified? Has Mrs Adams been able to understand and cooperate with all investigations?

NURSING PROBLEM 10.2

Problem: Mrs Adams needs to be taught how to carry out a 24-hour urine collection.
Goal: Mrs Adams will be able to carry out a 24-hour urine collection.

Intervention: 24-hour urine collection

A 24-hour urine collection may be required to determine the excretion of certain substances such as protein, glucose, and certain electrolytes and hormones.

This type of specimen may be collected at home or in hospital. To successfully collect the specimen, Mrs Adams needs to be provided with at least one labelled collection bottle, a receiver and a jug. She will also need easy access to a toilet.

Mrs Adams will need to be instructed as follows:

● When the collection is started, Mrs Adams should discard the first sample. The time this sample was passed should be noted on the specimen container. This is the starting time for the collection.

- After this, every time she passes urine it should be poured into the container.
- At the end of the 24-hour period, at the same time as it was started, she should empty her bladder and include this in the collection.
- The specimen label should then be completed to record finishing time.
- The specimen should be kept cool before being transported to the laboratory.
- All urine must be saved throughout the 24-hour period. If Mrs Adams fails to do this, the sample should be discarded and re-commenced.
- Mrs Adams should be given these instructions in writing.

Evaluation

Did Mrs Adams manage to collect a 24-hour sample without any problems?

Care of a patient with a urinary catheter

Patients who have a urinary catheter inserted as part of their care are at risk of developing a catheter-related infection in the following situations (Baillie and Arrowsmith 2001):

- obstruction of the normal closing mechanism of the bladder by the catheter
- the loss of natural flushing of the urethra through passing urine
- in women, catheters are situated near the anus, which may lead to the transfer of bowel organisms to the urinary tract
- if drainage tubing or catheter becomes kinked, it may result in a backflow of urine to the ureters or kidneys which may cause pyelonephritis
- cross-infection, which may be introduced if infection control guidelines are not followed.

NURSING PROBLEM 10.3

Patient history: Mrs Holder had a urinary catheter inserted during abdominal surgery.

Problem: Mrs Holder is at risk of acquiring an infection of the urethra and bladder as she has a urinary catheter in situ following surgery.

Goal: Mrs Holder will not develop an infection of the urethra and bladder.

Intervention: daily perineal cleansing

If Mrs Holder is able, she should be encouraged to carry out daily perineal cleansing herself, since it will both reduce the risk of cross-infection and help to preserve her dignity. If this is not possible, the nurse should assist or do it for her. If Mrs Holder is able to perform self-care, she should follow the same guidelines detailed below, with the exception of applying gloves and an apron.

Equipment

- Soap.
- Warm water.
- Disposable wipes.
- Clean towel.
- Towel and plastic sheet to protect bed linen.

Procedure

- Explain procedure to Mrs Holder.
- Prepare equipment.

TIP! Some literature advocates the use of special solutions for perineal/ meatal cleansing but the use of soap and warm water with clean wipes has been shown to be equally effective in preventing infection (Wilson 1997).

- Provide privacy by drawing the curtains and closing the door.
- Assist Mrs Holder to adopt a supine position with knees and hips flexed and slightly apart. Place towel and plastic sheet under her bottom and thighs.
- Wash and dry your hands. Put on apron and gloves.
- Using soap, warm water and clean disposable wipes, clean the perineal area by wiping from front to back to reduce risk of transfer of micro-organisms from the bowel to the catheter entry into the meatus (catheter–meatal junction). Each cloth should be used just once to prevent transfer of micro-organisms.
- Clean the catheter by wiping in one direction away from the vulva.
- Dry Mrs Holder by patting with a clean towel. Avoid applying powders and lotions as these may trap organisms in the area (Nicol et al. 2000).
- Help Mrs Holder to assume a comfortable position.
- Dispose of waste.
- Remove gloves and apron.
- Wash and dry hands.
- Document care provided and report any abnormalities to senior colleagues.

TIP! To perform meatal cleansing, male patients should retract the foreskin and clean away from the catheter–meatal junction, using soap, warm water and disposable cloths. The area should be rinsed well and dried with a clean towel. The foreskin should then be replaced.

Intervention: emptying urinary catheter drainage bag

Micro-organisms can easily ascend to the bladder by entering the drainage tap that empties the catheter bag. It is therefore vital that the infection control guidelines are followed when emptying catheter bags.

Equipment

- Non-sterile gloves.
- Apron.

- Disinfected or disposable receiver.
- Cover for receiver.
- Two alcohol swabs.

Procedure

- Prepare equipment.
- Explain the procedure to Mrs Holder.
- Screen the bed if Mrs Holder requests this or if she needs to be exposed in order to allow access to the drainage bag.
- Wash and dry hands and put on gloves and apron.
- Clean the outlet tap of the bag with an alcohol swab and allow it to dry.
- Open the tap allowing the urine to drain into the receiver. Ensure that the tap does not touch the receiver or the floor and that your gloved fingers do not touch the exit point.
- Close the tap and wipe it with the second alcohol swab.
- Position the bag so that it does not touch the floor and is in a comfortable and discreet position.
- Cover the receiver, take it to the sluice and, if required, measure the urine.
- Dispose of urine and disinfect or dispose of receiver as per local policy.
- Remove gloves and apron.
- Wash and dry hands.
- Document volume on fluid balance chart if required.
- Report any abnormalities in odour, volume, colour or consistency of urine to a senior colleague.

Intervention: avoid unnecessary changes of catheter bags and drainage tubing

Micro-organisms can easily enter the bladder via the junction between the catheter and drainage tubing. Unnecessary changes or disconnections in the closed drainage system, catheter bags and drainage tubing should therefore be avoided.

Intervention: drainage bag position

Position the drainage bag below the level of the bladder and clear of potential sources of contamination to facilitate drainage. The use of a catheter bag stand will prevent contact of the port with the floor, thus reducing the risk of infection. The patient will appreciate discreet placement of the bag beside the bed or when mobilizing to maintain her dignity.

Intervention: prevent kinks in the catheter and drainage tubing

Kinks in the catheter and drainage tubing may result in a backflow of urine to the ureters or kidneys, which may cause infection. It also causes stagnation of urine in the drainage tube which may encourage bacterial growth.

Intervention: anchor the catheter to Mrs Holder's thigh

Evidence suggests that this may reduce infection in females, as movement of the catheter can lead to ascending infection due to the short length of the female urethra (Ayliffe et al. 1999).

Intervention: increase fluid intake to 2–3 litres per day

Advise Mrs Holder to increase her fluid intake to more than 2 litres per day if her condition permits. This will result in an increased flow of urine through the drainage system which makes it more difficult for bacteria to ascend to the bladder (Baillie and Arrowsmith 2001) or to multiply in the bladder.

Intervention: removal of urinary catheter

A urine catheter may be removed when:

- no longer required
- to be replaced with a new one
- if urine is not flowing freely and all attempts to clear a blockage are unsuccessful
- urine is bypassing the catheter, causing leakage.

Catheters should be removed as soon as possible, as the risk of infection increases with each additional day that they are in situ (Wilson 1995). Alternatives to long-term catheterization, such as supra-pubic catheters, or intermittent self-catheterization, may be used in some instances to reduce complications. Evidence suggests that removing a catheter at midnight (Noble et al. 1990), or last thing at night, improves return to normal bladder function.

Explain that after removal there may be some feelings of urgency when passing water. Mrs Holder may also experience frequency and some discomfort, with possible haematuria (blood-stained urine) following removal. Ensure that toilet facilities are close by, and ask Mrs Holder to report when she has managed to pass urine after the catheter is removed.

Equipment

- Receiver.
- 10 ml syringe.
- Disposable waterproof pad.
- Clinical waste bag.
- Specimen pot, needle and syringe for CSU if required (see page 250).
- Gauze swabs or tissues.
- Apron and gloves.

Procedure

- Explain the procedure to Mrs Holder.
- Check Mrs Holder's notes to verify how much water was put into the balloon on insertion of the catheter.
- Wash hands.
- Gather equipment and place on clean tray.
- Draw the curtains and assist Mrs Holder to adopt a supine position with knees and hips flexed and slightly apart. Protect her dignity and keep her warm with a blanket.
- Wash and dry your hands. Put on apron and gloves.
- Obtain a CSU if needed.
- Place absorbent sheet under Mrs Holder's bottom and thighs, and place receiver between her thighs.
- Attach syringe to balloon port of the catheter and slowly withdraw full amount of water.
- When Mrs Holder is ready, ask her to inhale and exhale deeply. As she exhales, gently withdraw the catheter and place it in the receiver. She may experience feelings of wanting to pass urine at once, but encourage her to wait until the feeling passes off.

Tightening of the pelvic muscles as if stopping the flow of urine in mid-stream can reduce this feeling.

ALERT!

If any resistance is felt or if bleeding occurs stop and seek advice from a senior colleague or doctor.

- Wash Mrs Holder's skin if urine has spilt onto it and change her bed if necessary.
- Help Mrs Holder to assume a comfortable position and open the screens around the bed.
- Take waste to the sluice and measure urine volume if required.
- Dispose of urine and equipment, adhering to infection control policies.
- Remove gloves and apron.
- Wash and dry hands.
- Ensure that a toilet or commode is nearby, or a call bell if assistance is required.
- Document catheter removal and volume of urine, if required.
- Monitor urine output and observe for dysuria (pain on voiding) and haematuria (blood in urine). Advise Mrs Holder to maintain an oral fluid intake of more than 2 litres in 24 hours.

Intervention: obtaining a CSU

In certain Trusts, a CSU is routinely obtained on removal of the catheter to check for the presence of infection.

Equipment

- Alcohol swab.
- 10 ml syringe.
- Needle (if required – use size recommended by manufacturer).
- Sterile specimen container.
- Pathology request form.
- Gate clamp.

Procedure

- Explain the procedure to Mrs Holder, and provide privacy.
- Prepare equipment.

- Wash and dry your hands. Put on apron and gloves.
- Locate sample port on catheter bag tubing. This may be a latex port, which requires a needle and syringe to obtain a sample, or a needleless port that requires only a syringe.
- If there is no urine present in the tubing, clamp the tube below the port until there is a sufficient quantity.
- Swab the sample port with an alcohol swab and allow the port to dry.
- If a needle is required to obtain the sample, attach this to the syringe and insert it at a 45° angle to reduce the risk of the needle going through the tubing. If the port is a needleless system, attach the syringe to it.
- Aspirate sample.
- Remove clamp (if used). Remove needle from the syringe and dispose of in sharps box.
- Transfer the sample into the sterile specimen pot.
- Label the container clearly with Mrs Holder's name, identity number/address, date of birth, date and time collected and examination required. Place in plastic specimen bag.
- Place specimen in refrigerator and ensure that it is transported to the laboratory promptly.
- Remove gloves and apron.
- Wash hands.
- Document collection of specimen in Mrs Holder's notes.

Evaluation

Was a positive result obtained from the CSU? Signs of infection may include pyrexia, offensive urine and abdominal discomfort, and will indicate the need to reassess Mrs Holder's care.

NURSING PROBLEM 10.4

Patient history: Mrs Bright is an elderly lady who has recently had a stroke. She needs assistance with most activities of living due to a residual left-sided weakness.

Problem: Mrs Bright is unable to toilet herself unaided.

Goal: Mrs Bright will state that her toileting needs have been met and her dignity maintained.

Assistance with toileting

The following principles (Baillie and Arrowsmith 2001) should be taken into consideration when assisting patients to use the toilet, commode, bedpan or urinal:

- The ability to anticipate patients' elimination needs and to be responsive to communication signals from patients. For example, nonverbal cues such as restlessness may need to be recognized for patients with communication difficulties.
- Provision of privacy and dignity.
- Prompt response to requests for assistance with toileting.
- Maintenance of infection control principles.
- Observation of the patient's skin, output, mobility and cognitive function when assisting the patient.
- Anticipation of risks and prevention of accidents.
- Promotion of patient independence and participation.
- Hygiene and comfort should be a priority.

When assisting with toileting, it is important to assess the degree of independence that the patient retains so that dignity and independence can be promoted. For many patients, the last time anyone assisted them in the toilet was when they were small children, and they may find the activity demeaning if not approached sensitively by the nurse. The sights, sounds and smells that accompany elimination activities are usually considered to be very personal, and patients may be distressed on occasions if they are not able to maintain their usual routine or if they feel they are being overheard. Some cultural practices may not be easily followed if there is an attendant in the toilet, and an awareness of particular cultural needs is necessary. For example, some cultures consider the left hand as unclean and use it for all elimination purposes, whilst retaining the right hand for eating purposes only, thus requiring the availability of running water for cleaning after toileting to maintain their usual habits.

TIP! **The terms used to ask for toilet facilities vary between generations and localities. An elderly person requesting a 'visit to her aunt' or a chance to 'spend a penny' may not indicate confusion or a desire to take a walk, but the desire to go to the** lavatory. **If you are new to an area, try to find out what the local terms are for toilet facilities so that you can respond quickly and without embarrassing the patient.**

Intervention: assisting with toileting needs

Whenever possible, a person should be encouraged to use the toilet since the bathroom provides privacy and is a familiar environment for elimination. Mrs Bright may need assistance with walking to the toilet or she may need to use a wheelchair and be assisted to transfer on to the toilet. She may also need assistance with unbuttoning or unzipping her clothes, removing undergarments, wiping herself, getting dressed and handwashing. It is the nurse's role to provide this assistance. Patients may be embarrassed to ask for such intimate help, but dignity can be preserved if the nurse shows respect and understanding.

To prevent cross-infection, the nurse should wear non-sterile gloves and an apron whilst helping Mrs Bright to clean herself. Manual handling guidelines should be adhered to when assisting Mrs Bright to transfer to the toilet or to walk.

Intervention: assistance with using a commode

If Mrs Bright is too weak to mobilize to the toilet but is able to get out of bed, a commode is preferable to using a bedpan since it is more comfortable and allows a better position for elimination without undue strain. If Mrs Bright requires frequent access to the commode, it may be appropriate to nurse her in a single room to aid privacy.

Equipment

- Commode containing clean bedpan.
- Cover.
- Toilet paper.
- Hand-cleansing wipes or soap, water and towel.
- Gloves and apron.

Procedure

- Explain the procedure to Mrs Bright.
- Prepare equipment.

- Prepare any manual handling aids and ask for assistance as required to ensure a safe transfer from bed to commode.
- Close the room door and screen off bed area.
- Place commode next to bed, allowing sufficient space for Mrs Bright to transfer safely. Apply brakes.
- Check that the bed brakes are on and adjust the height of the bed to facilitate a safe transfer.
- Help Mrs Bright to put on her slippers and dressing gown.
- Assist Mrs Bright as required to transfer to the commode. Help her to undress and then sit down on the commode.
- If Mrs Bright is frail, move the commode so that she can lean on the edge of the bed.
- If Mrs Bright's condition allows, leave her alone to provide privacy but provide her with the call bell and remain nearby.
- When Mrs Bright is ready assist her with cleansing as required. Gloves and an apron should be worn for this aspect of the procedure.
- Assist Mrs Bright to return to bed or chair and help her to wash her hands.
- Dispose of excreta, clean/macerate bedpan and clean commode as per local policy.
- Remove gloves and apron. Wash hands.
- Document bowel action and/or urinary output.

TIP! **Commodes should have their seat and handrests wiped between patients to prevent cross-infection.**

Intervention: assistance with using a bedpan

Mrs Bright may be unable to get out of bed in which case a bedpan will need to be used. There are two types of bedpan: a standard bedpan which requires the bottom to be lifted up in order to get onto it, or a flat 'slipper' pan which can be rolled onto (Figure 10.2.1). Bedpans may be reusable or disposable. Reusable pans (Figure 10.2.2) must be washed thoroughly in a washer-disinfector that has been designed for this purpose and is regularly maintained. Disposable bedpans (Figure 10.2.3) are usually disposed of using a macerator. These bedpans are made out of paper pulp; they therefore need to be used inside a plastic support which should be cleaned as per local policy after use.

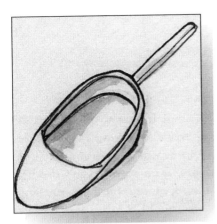

Figure 10.2.1
Slipper pan.

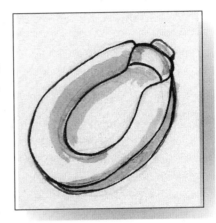

Figure 10.2.2
Reusable pan.

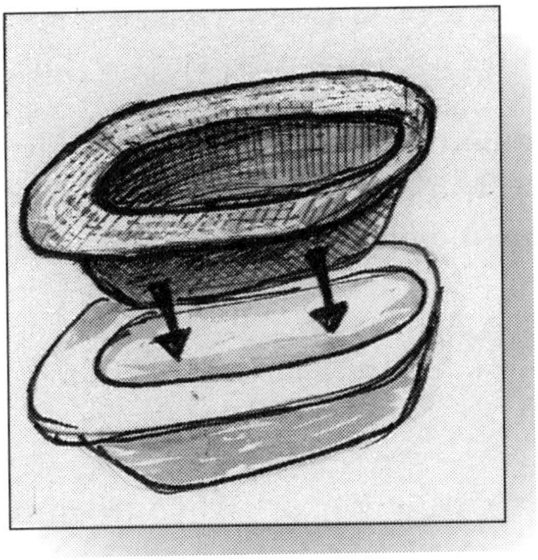

Figure 10.2.3
Disposable pan
with plastic
support.

Figure 10.2.1–3 Bedpans.

Equipment

- Bedpan and cover.
- Toilet paper.
- Hand-cleansing wipes or soap, water and towel.
- Gloves and apron.

Procedure

- Assess which type of bedpan is required.
- Explain the procedure to Mrs Bright.
- Prepare equipment.

TIP! If using a metal bedpan, the patient may find it cold to sit on and that will discourage her from emptying her bladder. Warming the pan with warm tap water and drying it thoroughly will help to overcome this, *but* be careful with the hot water or you may overheat the bedpan and burn the patient! It should be warm, but not hot, to touch.

- Prepare any manual handling aids and ask for as much assistance as required to assist Mrs Bright in getting onto the bedpan safely.
- Provide privacy by drawing the curtains.
- Ask Mrs Bright to raise her bottom and place the wide rim of the bedpan underneath her buttocks with the narrow area situated between the legs. If using a slipper bedpan, help Mrs Bright to roll to one side, place the pan under her pelvis with the handle positioned towards the legs and assist her to roll back onto the pan.

TIP! Patients who are confined to bed and who are able to lift themselves using a hoist should use this to lift themselves up so that the bedpan can be slipped under them.

- Cover Mrs Bright with bedding and leave her alone to provide privacy but leave her with the call bell and remain nearby. Ensure she has toilet paper to hand.

TIP! Females need to have their legs slightly apart when using a bedpan, otherwise urine may travel down the legs. Males may prefer to either urinate into a urinal or position the penis downwards into the bedpan to prevent spillage.
If a patient has difficulty passing urine the sound of a running tap may help.

- When Mrs Bright is ready, assist her with cleansing as required and remove the bedpan. Gloves and an apron should be worn for this aspect of the procedure. The bedpan may be placed on a chair or stool while you make Mrs Bright comfortable. Placing it on the floor will collect additional micro-organisms and increase infection risks.

TIP! If patients need assistance with cleansing following defaecation, disposable cloths and warm water or wet wipes may be acceptable. The perineal area should be wiped with disposable tissue or cloths from front to back to discourage faecal organisms from entering the urine tract. Ensure the skin is left clean and dry.

- Straighten Mrs Bright's sheets and help her into a comfortable position.
- Help Mrs Bright to clean her hands.
- Dispose of excreta, clean/macerate bedpan and clean bedpan holder as per local policy.
- Remove gloves and apron.
- Wash hands.
- Document bowel action and/or urinary output.

TIP! If assisting a lady who is menstruating to use a bedpan or commode, provide a sanitary towel disposal bag and clean sanitary protection. She may also appreciate a bowl of warm water and washing equipment if there has been menstrual leakage. Be prepared to assist with this if necessary.

Evaluation

Has Mrs Bright been able to use the bedpan comfortably? Have spillages been avoided, indicating that the appropriate sort of bedpan is being offered?

NURSING PROBLEM 10.5

Patient history: Mr Solomon has limited mobility and cannot get out to the toilet without assistance. Sometimes he suffers from urinary dribbling and incontinence, especially at night.

Problem: Mr Solomon needs assistance with toileting.

Goal: Mr Solomon will be able to retain urinary continence.

Assistance with male urination

Male patients have the advantage of being able to use a urinal to pass water. Urinals may be plastic, glass or disposable.

Intervention: to assist Mr Solomon to use the urinal

- Collect the urinal, urinal holder and disposable cover and take it to Mr Solomon.
- Show Mr Solomon the urinal and explain its use.
- Place the urinal in the holder and place on the side of the bed nearest to Mr Solomon's dominant hand so that he can reach it easily.

TIP! Urinals tend to be placed on patients' bed tables for ease of access, but this is unhygienic, and should be discouraged. It could put a patient off his food and contaminate other articles on the table. Make sure urinals are positioned discreetly but within the patient's reach. Tell him where you have put it so it can be found easily.

- If Mr Solomon needs help to use the urinal, draw the curtains to provide privacy, and put on gloves and apron.
- Lift the bedcovers and open the pyjama bottoms to expose the penis. If Mr Solomon is able, encourage him to place his penis into the urinal. Ensure that the urinal is placed with the bottom end downwards otherwise there will be backflow and the bed will get wet. Patients may find this very distressing as they think that they have been incontinent.

TIP! Some men, particularly after operations, find it very difficult to pass water lying down, and may prefer to stand to pass water. They can lean with their bottom on the bed. Ensure the brakes are applied, and if the patient is rather unsteady provide support from two nurses.

- When Mr Solomon has finished, remove his penis from the urinal, shaking it a little if necessary to remove any drips. Place disposable cover over the urinal, and place into the holder.
- Assist Mr Solomon to adjust his clothing and make him comfortable.

TIP! Patients with dribbling incontinence may be keen to keep a urinal in place all the time, but this may cause the penis to be in a constantly damp environment and cause skin maceration. Encourage regular and frequent toileting instead.

- Empty the urinal, recording amount if required, and taking note of the consistency, colour and odour of the urine.
- Document as necessary and report any abnormalities to senior staff.
- Replace the used urinal with a fresh one.

TIP! Many men are able to use a urinal without assistance, but will need a fresh one provided at regular intervals during the day. Overfull urinals may get knocked over and spilt so offer to change it during every shift.

Intervention: application of a penile sheath

If Mr Solomon finds that he cannot use a urinal effectively, he may prefer to have a penile sheath fitted. Penile sheaths are fitted onto the penis allowing urine to be channelled into a collection bag (Figure 10.3). They are useful for men with urinary incontinence and for men who experience frequency and urgency but are unable to get to the toilet easily.

TIP! Silicone sheaths are available for people with latex allergy.

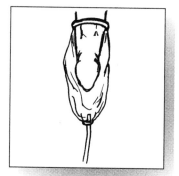

Figure 10.3.1
Penile sheath.

Figure 10.3.2
Sheath
draining into
leg bag.

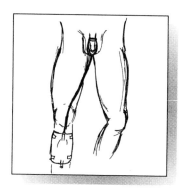

Figure 10.3.1–2 Application of penile sheath and leg bag.

Both clear and opaque sheaths are available. An opaque sheath may be more acceptable to the patient, but clear sheaths allow clear observation of the penile skin.

Equipment

- Assortment of sheaths with adhesive in different sizes.
- Catheter drainage bag.
- Disposable tape measure.
- Gloves and apron.
- Soap, warm water, disposable wipes and towel.

Procedure

- Explain procedure to Mr Solomon.
- Prepare equipment.

- Provide privacy by drawing the curtains.
- Assist Mr Solomon to sit up in bed.
- Put on gloves and apron.
- Ask or assist Mr Solomon to wash and dry penis and surrounding area.
- Measure circumference of penis at its widest point and measure length using a disposable tape measure.
- Select appropriately sized sheath.
- Trim pubic hair at base of penis if required.
- If using a two-part sheath instruct Mr Solomon to apply the adhesive strip to the shaft of the penis. Care should be taken to avoid a tourniquet effect, by positioning the adhesive in a spiral fashion.
- Fit the sheath, or instruct Mr Solomon to roll it over the penis, starting at the tip and rolling it down the shaft. Leave a space between end of penis and cup of sheath to allow for expansion of penis. If Mr Solomon is not circumcised do not retract the fore-skin.
- Attach to a urine collection bag.
- Ensure that Mr Solomon is comfortable.
- Remove gloves and apron.
- Wash hands.
- Document actions and condition of penile skin in Mr Solomon's notes.

Evaluation

Has Mr Solomon retained continence? Has the penile sheath been effective in collecting urine and keeping him dry and comfortable?

NURSING PROBLEM 10.6

Problem: Mr Solomon has limited mobility and therefore he is at risk of developing constipation.

Goal: Mr Solomon will maintain or return to his normal bowel pattern.

Constipation

Constipation can be defined as fewer than three bowel movements a week, though additional symptoms like straining, passing hard stools and the inability to defaecate when desired, together with abdominal pain, form part of the diagnosis (Bandolier 1997).

Patients commonly complain of constipation, but they may think they are constipated because they have not had a daily bowel motion. As can be seen from the definition, infrequency of defaecation alone is not an indication of constipation, and may in fact have other causes such as changes in lifestyle or environment. Many people experience constipation when away from home but their normal bowel habit resumes on their return home. Elderly patients may present only with increased confusion and very few other obvious symptoms, so constipation is worth considering in such circumstances.

The cause of constipation needs to be determined and therefore it is important to take a history. Important questions to ask are:

- What are the normal bowel habits and frequency of defaecation?
- Is there any associated abdominal bloating or flatus?
- How long have they been experiencing these symptoms? When did they start?
- What kind of stool is passed? E.g. is it hard, soft, small or large?
- How much fibre and fluids are normally taken in the diet?
- Is there any associated pain, straining or urgency?
- Have there been any recent changes in lifestyle or environment?
- What type of medications are normally taken? This includes medications that may induce constipation and also any regular medication that the patient may take to prevent constipation.

The history will probably identify that the patient is experiencing infrequent, painful and difficult defaecation, possibly associated with straining to empty the bowel, and a feeling of incomplete emptying. There may be some soiling of clothes, which indicates faecal impaction with faecal overflow, which can be mistaken for diarrhoea. There may be associated abdominal pain or bloating, and a general feeling of malaise, headache and bad taste in the mouth (Kamm and Lennard

Jones 1994). The history may also find a relationship with one of the following five areas:

- Mode of life – there may be inadequate dietary fibre or fluid taken, a reduced intake of food, a repressed response to the urge to open bowels, or reduced mobility.
- External factors – these include drugs such as opiates, antidepressants, and anticholinergics. Having to use a bedpan in hospital, the experience of inadequate privacy, and inadequate pain relief also contribute.
- Endocrine or metabolic disorders – e.g. hypothyroidism.
- Neurological – e.g. Parkinson's disease, multiple sclerosis.
- Psychological – e.g. depression or anorexia nervosa.

Intervention: prevention of constipation

- Record frequency, appearance and consistency of Mr Solomon's bowel movements. This allows monitoring and recording of effectiveness of any preventative interventions that have been instigated.
- Encourage a high fibre diet and increased fluid intake. Bran and high fibre foods have been shown to work as effectively as regular laxatives (Bandolier 1997). Patients who are immobile tend to have a slower passage of food through the gut and additional fibre and fluids encourages the maintenance of a soft and regular stool.
- Assist Mr Solomon to the toilet after meals and allow him to sit for a short time to facilitate the gastro-colic reflex. Where patients have limited mobility this has been found to encourage a natural response to the urge to defaecate (Getliffe and Dolman 1997).
- Provide privacy and encourage the use of commode or toilet rather than a bedpan, to provide a conducive environment and a natural position for defaecation.
- If medication likely to induce constipation is in use, e.g. opiates, ensure that an appropriate preventative laxative is also prescribed. Follow local guidelines as to prescription and use of laxatives, enemas and suppositories.

NURSING PROBLEM 10.7

Patient history: Mr Campbell has been on the ward for several days for investigations. Today he is complaining of diarrhoea.
Problem: Mr Campbell is passing unformed, offensive stools.
Goal: To detect underlying cause within x days.

Diarrhoea

Diarrhoea is usually related to accelerated movement of contents through the intestine in addition to a decrease in mixing and absorption, resulting in frequent liquid or unformed stools.

Diarrhoea is associated with many bowel disorders as well as other disorders that are not associated with the intestine. Intrinsic causes include:

- diverticulitis
- faecal impaction with overflow
- laxatives
- infection
- neoplasms
- dietary changes
- antibiotics.

Extrinsic causes include:

- emotional stress
- systemic disorders such as acute infectious disease and uraemia.

A detailed history is therefore essential in helping to identify the underlying cause.

Intervention: obtain a detailed history

Information needs to be obtained regarding:

- the nature and onset of Mr Campbell's symptoms – frequency, amount, consistency, colour, pain, flatus
- usual eating patterns and responses to food
- past history of gastro-intestinal disorders
- medications (both prescribed and non-prescribed)
- usual patterns of bowel elimination
- any recent visits to a foreign country
- potential exposure to food poisoning
- any recent contact with individuals suffering similar symptoms
- presence of blood, parasites, mucus in stool
- recent constipation
- exposure to emotional stress.

Intervention: obtain a faecal specimen

Faecal specimens may be examined for blood, parasites, organisms and specific food residues such as fat.

Equipment

- Bedpan.
- Toilet tissue.
- Sterile stool specimen pot with spoon attached to lid, or a sterile universal container and spatula.
- Specimen bag.
- Laboratory request form.
- Gloves and apron.

Procedure

- Explain procedure to Mr Campbell.
- Prepare equipment.
- Instruct Mr Campbell to place bedpan inside the toilet seat to obtain the specimen.

TIP! To make it easier to collect a specimen of loose stool, before the bedpan is used place plenty of toilet roll into it to soak up any urine.

- When specimen is ready, put on gloves and apron. Cover specimen and take to sluice.
- Uncover specimen and use spoon in lid of container or the spatula to collect a small quantity of faeces. Place this in the sterile container and secure the lid.
- Label the container clearly with Mr Campbell's name, identity number/address, date of birth, date and time collected and examination required. Place in plastic specimen bag.
- Dispose of excreta, bedpan and spatula as per local policy.
- Remove gloves and apron.
- Wash hands.
- Place specimen in refrigerator and ensure that it is transported to the laboratory promptly. If the test is for parasites, the specimen must be kept warm and delivered to the laboratory immediately.
- Document collection of specimen in Mr Campbell's notes. Report the presence of blood, excessive mucus, or parasites.

Intervention: prepare Mr Campbell for any further investigations

Further investigations may include:

- examination of abdomen for palpable mass
- rectal examination to exclude faecal impaction
- blood tests to examine blood chemistry, electrolytes, haematological profile and blood cultures
- computerized axial tomography
- endoscopy
- colonoscopy, sigmoidoscopy and proctoscopy.

Psychological preparation for these tests will include a full explanation of the investigation and the care required both before and after the procedure. Mr Campbell should be given written information about the investigation and every opportunity to ask questions should be offered. Physical preparation should reflect local protocols.

Evaluation

Was the cause of diarrhoea identified from the sample and history? Was Mr Campbell able to cooperate with all investigations?

Stoma appliances

The word 'stoma' refers to an 'artificial opening'. When surgery is required to remove part of the bowel or bladder as a result of disease or trauma, a stoma is formed on the surface of the abdomen to allow excretion of faecal matter or urine.

A 'colostomy' is an artificial opening of the colon onto the abdominal surface. It may originate from:

- the sigmoid colon
- the descending colon
- the transverse colon
- the ascending colon.

A colostomy is usually sited at the left iliac fossa. If the colostomy exits from the sigmoid or descending colon, its output will be formed with a normal faecal odour. If it is sited in the transverse or ascending colon, the output will be loose and copious with a strong odour.

An 'ileostomy' is an artificial opening of the ileum onto the abdominal surface. It is usually sited in the right iliac fossa. The output from an ileostomy ('effluent') is very soft and fluid, which necessitates emptying of the appliance approximately six times per day.

A 'urostomy' is formed when the bladder is removed ('cystectomy') and a urinary diversion is raised in the form of a stoma.

Information about appliances

In the initial post-operative period, a clear plastic appliance (stoma pouch) is used to allow observation of output. However, opaque appliances may be used later. Colostomy bags are available with flatus filters and charcoal filters to decrease odour. A patient with an ileostomy will need to use a drainable device, where the end is sealed with a tie or plastic clip. These are also available with filters. Urostomy appliances have a tap at the bottom to allow frequent drainage and connection to an overnight collection bag. Urostomy bags have a non-reflux valve inside to prevent urine flowing back up to the stoma which may cause skin soreness and leakage.

NURSING PROBLEM 10.8

Patient history: Mrs McCarthy has had a new colostomy formed in her left iliac fossa. She is to start learning how to care for it herself to prepare for discharge.

Problem: Mrs McCarthy is unable to change her stoma appliance.

Goal: Mrs McCarthy will be able to change her stoma appliance prior to discharge from hospital.

Care of stoma appliances

The following interventions will help Mrs McCarthy learn how to change her stoma appliance. First, however, it is important to assess whether Mrs McCarthy is ready to learn the procedure.

Although the development of practical skills in caring for her stoma will enable Mrs McCarthy to regain some independence, she may become demoralized if a teaching programme is commenced before she is emotionally prepared.

Many patients feel extremely traumatized following surgery for the formation of a stoma. Altered body image, perceived physical mutilation, loss of control over bladder or bowel function, and fear as to whether she will ever be able to care for her own stoma may result in Mrs McCarthy feeling overwhelmed and anxious (Metcalf 1999). It is essential that these issues are addressed before embarking on teaching Mrs McCarthy how to care for her stoma, since they are likely to prevent her from learning (Thomson 1988). In addition, any physical or cognitive impairments must be considered before embarking on a teaching programme.

Additional care and help would be required for Mrs McCarthy if assessment suggests that Mrs McCarthy is struggling to come to terms with her stoma.

When Mrs McCarthy is ready introduce her to the procedure. As she gains confidence encourage her to participate in changing her stoma bag. A particularly effective method of teaching practical skills is to demonstrate the entire procedure first, explaining what you are doing throughout. The procedure is then broken down into component parts (see below) and the patient learns each part at her own pace. Learning how to change a stoma bag in the bathroom setting will help prepare Mrs McCarthy for discharge as it is more realistic to the home situation. The bathroom also provides privacy.

TIP! It is useful to have a mirror available to check for correct application of the appliance.

Intervention: changing a stoma bag

The procedure for changing a stoma bag which is detailed below has been written for Mrs McCarthy to perform. However, if the nurse is performing the procedure, gloves and an apron should be worn.

Equipment

- Warm water in sink.
- Soft wipes/gauze (not tissue or toilet paper as this disintegrates when wet).
- New appliance.
- Scissors.
- Template.
- Clip or tie fixed on bottom of pouch if required.
- Plastic disposal bag.
- Protective sheet/tissue paper.
- Pen.
- Barrier cream if advised.
- Gloves and apron if nurse assists.

Procedure

- Prepare equipment.
- Protect clothing.
- If Mrs McCarthy is wearing a drainable pouch she should empty it first (see below) to avoid spillage.
- Remove soiled pouch by starting at the top of the flange and gently peeling from top to bottom. Use the free hand to support surrounding skin.

- Wash around stoma and surrounding skin using soft wipes. Place these in rubbish bag.
- Thoroughly dry skin with soft wipes. Dispose of wipes.
- Check the condition of the stoma and surrounding skin and apply barrier cream if advised.
- If necessary, measure the size of the stoma and make a template. Using the template cut the flange to the correct size. The flange should fit snugly around the stoma. If it is too small, the edge of the flange may cause bruising or bleeding due to friction with the stoma. If it is too big, excrement may spill onto the surrounding skin causing soreness and, potentially, skin breakdown.
- Remove backing paper from the new stoma bag. Fold the bag in half so that the flange is rounded. Position the bag onto the stoma by matching lower edge of opening with bottom edge of stoma. Fold top half of the flange over stoma and press firmly on the skin. Ensure that the stoma mucosa is not covered with the flange.
- Apply gentle pressure around the flange ensuring that it adheres to the skin. Check that it is free of creases as these may cause leakage.
- Empty soiled pouch into toilet and discard into rubbish bag.
- Wash hands.
- Document how Mrs McCarthy coped with the procedure and that the stoma bag has been changed. Any problems should be reported to a senior colleague.

TIP! **Different councils and health authorities have different regulations concerning the disposal of clinical waste in the community. Mrs McCarthy will need to be taught how to adhere to the regulations for her particular area.**

Intervention: emptying a drainable pouch

If Mrs McCarthy uses a drainable pouch, she will also need to learn how to empty this. The procedure for doing this, which is detailed below, has been written for Mrs McCarthy to perform. However, if the nurse is performing the procedure, gloves and an apron should be worn.

Equipment

- A receiver.
- Protective sheet/tissue for clothing.

- Tissue paper.
- Plastic bag for waste.
- Gloves and apron if nurse assists.

Procedure

- Prepare equipment.
- Protect clothing.
- Place receiver under outlet of pouch.
- Remove clip/open tap at end of pouch.
- Empty pouch contents into container.
- Clean outlet of pouch with tissue, going at least one inch inside the bag. (This is not necessary with a urostomy bag.)
- Apply cleaned clip.
- Dispose of waste according to local policy.

Evaluation

Can Mrs McCarthy state that she can change her own pouch? Does she appear confident and able to care for it herself? Is the stoma nurse confident that Mrs McCarthy has mastered the technique to care for her stoma?

Intervention: discharging a patient with a stoma

Prior to discharge it is *essential* that the following issues are addressed:

- Follow-up by the GP, District Nurse and Community Stoma Care Nurse must be arranged so that Mrs McCarthy can be helped with any potential problems: e.g. difficulty in adapting and coping; stoma retraction; sore skin; peristomal hernia; prolapse; and stenosis (Black 2000).
- Mrs McCarthy must be made aware of any specific nutritional requirements, such as changes to her diet to affect faecal output (Black 2000).
- In preparation for discharge, obtain sufficient supplies for the patient to be able to take home a week's supply of equipment.
- Mrs McCarthy should be given contact numbers for the Hospital and Community Stoma Care Nurses, and details of local support groups.

Assisting patients with nausea and vomiting

Nausea is an unpleasant and sometimes distressing symptom in which one feels the inclination to vomit. It is usually accompanied by discomfort in the abdominal region, hypersalivation, with sweating or feeling hot and cold. It may or may not lead to vomiting. Vomiting is the ejection of gastric contents. It is usually preceded by nausea although not always.

Nausea and vomiting are very common symptoms and are associated with a wide range of conditions including surgery, particularly when the gut has been handled. It is important to note, however, that surgery does not always cause these symptoms.

NURSING PROBLEM 10.9

Patient history: Mrs Child is recovering from an anaesthetic.
Problem: Mrs Child is experiencing post-operative nausea and vomiting.
Goals: Mrs Child will not aspirate her vomit.
Minimize Mrs Child's discomfort.

Intervention: preventing aspiration of vomit

Mrs Child may be drowsy following anaesthesia, and she is therefore at risk of aspiration. The following interventions will help to prevent this.

- Position Mrs Child on her side to facilitate the drainage of vomit from her mouth.
- Remove dentures if they are loose.
- Position the suction machine with a Yankuer sucker ready near to Mrs Child so that vomit can be removed from the mouth if necessary (see Chapter 8).
- Remain with Mrs Child when she is vomiting, hold a receiver beside her mouth and encourage her to vomit into it.

- Administer anti-emetic drugs as prescribed and monitor their effect.
- Reassure Mrs Child, explaining all procedures and interventions, since anxiety may exacerbate the problem.

Evaluation

Has Mrs Child's airway been maintained?

Intervention: minimizing Mrs Child's discomfort

Interventions to help you achieve this goal include:

- All interventions above for preventing aspiration of vomit.
- Draw screens around bed area to provide privacy.
- Put on gloves and apron.
- Mrs Child may find it helpful to have her forehead supported by the nurse's hand when she is retching. If she has an abdominal wound, she will find it comforting to support it with her hands or a pillow.
- Cleanse Mrs Child's mouth and lips after each emesis. Offer a mouthwash or wipe with a moistened tissue.
- Dispose of the receiver promptly, ensuring a fresh one is beside Mrs Child should she start vomiting again before your return.
- Change soiled bedding and clothing as required.
- Encourage Mrs Child to take deep breaths as this can reduce nausea.
- Ensure that Mrs Child is able to rest, with minimal disturbance and noise.
- Advise Mrs Child to change position very slowly as nausea tends to increase with motion.
- Ventilate the room, and try to keep strong smells such as disinfectant or food out of the area.
- Leave a clean bowl and tissues, call bell and mouthwash within Mrs Child's reach.

TIP! **Cover the bowl with a paper towel, as this is less suggestive – memories of vomiting may induce further vomiting.**

- Limit Mrs Child's oral intake until she feels less nauseated. Keep to sips of water or ice only if fluids are permitted.
- Accurately record intake and output.

ALERT!

If vomiting is prolonged, Mrs Child may require intravenous fluids and gastric drainage via a nasogastric tube. It is essential that her fluid balance chart is accurately maintained to allow assessment as to whether these interventions are required.

Evaluation

Did these measures relieve Mrs Child's discomfort? Were anti-emetics effective?

Further reading

Black P (2000) Practical stoma care. Nursing Standard 14(41): 47–53.

Getliffe K, Dolman M (1997) Promoting Continence: a Clinical and Research Resource. London: Bailliere Tindall.

Metcalf C (1999) Stoma care: empowering patients through teaching practical skills. British Journal of Nursing 8(9): 593–600.

Sander R (1999) Promoting urinary continence in residential care. Nursing Standard 14(13–15): 49–53.

Thomas S (2000) New continence guidance. Primary Health Care 10(6): 20–21.

Thomson I (1998) Teaching the skills to cope with a stoma. Nursing Times 94(4): 55–56.

CHAPTER 11

Aseptic procedures

Barbara Workman

Aims and learning outcomes

This chapter discusses the principles of asepsis, and the application of those principles when undertaking aseptic procedures. By the end of the chapter you will be able to:

- outline the principles of aseptic precautions
- apply these principles to practical tasks of preparing a sterile field, using sterile gloves, and assisting other health care professionals during aseptic procedures
- change a dressing, and remove wound drains and skin closures
- follow guidelines to insert a urinary catheter.

The last two procedures will require supervision in practice until you are competent to undertake them independently.

Asepsis

Asepsis can be defined as 'the prevention of microbial contamination of living tissue or fluid or sterile materials by excluding, removing or killing micro-organisms' (Xavier 1999), the aim being to prevent infection. Aseptic technique is the collective term for methods used to maintain asepsis, and is designed to interrupt the routes of transmission of infection between the patient, staff, equipment and environment. It is the first line of defence against infection and is commonly practised wherever invasive procedures take place.

Asepsis is achieved by using sterilized equipment; a non-touch technique to avoid direct contact with the site; taking precautions to reduce airborne micro-organisms; thorough cleansing of the patient and his environment; and effective handwashing by health care personnel (Xavier 1999). There have been some variable aseptic practices noted between practitioners and within Trusts, often relying on tradition rather than logical application of aseptic principles, and not always supported by appropriate evidence (Rowley 2001). A framework to encourage a consistent approach to aseptic procedures has been suggested by Rowley (2001). When undertaking aseptic procedures these principles can be remembered by using the framework ANTT: Aseptic Non-Touch Technique (Rowley 2001):

Always wash hands effectively

Never contaminate key parts

Touch non-key parts with confidence

Take appropriate infective precautions

Sterilized equipment

When a patient's skin or mucous membrane is broken due to an invasive procedure, such as a surgical incision or an intramuscular injection, infection is able to bypass the body's natural defences. Therefore all equipment used to penetrate the body's natural defences should be sterilized before use. If equipment cannot be sterilized, then disinfection, which removes harmful micro-organisms, is used to prevent the transmission of infection. For example, a sterile catheter is used to empty the bladder, but hands cannot be sterilized and must be disinfected before inserting the catheter.

Trolleys are usually disinfected before commencing dressings or other aseptic procedures by daily cleaning with warm water and detergent, followed by thorough drying (Ayliffe et al. 1999), but unless trolleys are visibly contaminated or there is a local outbreak of infection, such as MRSA, cleaning between patients is not essential (Briggs et al. 1996).

All sterile packaging should be checked prior to use for:

- integrity
- evidence of sterility
- secure seals
- expiry date.

Pre-packaged lotions should be sterile, as should any dressings that are to come into contact with a wound. Multi-dose vials of lotions should only be used for one patient to prevent cross-contamination.

Non-touch technique

A non-touch technique has been developed to prevent contamination of the area from micro-organisms on the hands. Historically, forceps have been used in dressing procedures, but Bree-Williams and Waterman (1996) found that their use was often incorrect and confused. Evidence suggests that forceps can damage delicate tissues and be less effective when cleaning an area than a sterile gloved hand (Tomlinson 1987) or irrigation, and therefore the use of forceps in aseptic dressing procedures is declining, although for some delicate manipulative tasks, such as removing sutures, forceps are useful.

Non-touch technique also means that any equipment that is used in an aseptic procedure will remain sterile only when touched by another sterile object. For example, while a needle and syringe are assembled, the barrel of the syringe and the hub of the needle are non-key parts and can be touched by hand, but key parts of the equipment such as the needle remain sterile until used during the procedure. When preparing and using a sterile field, there should be careful placement of the sterile equipment so contamination is kept to the minimum (Figure 11.1).

Implements such as forceps and syringes should be placed so that the area to be handled is at the edge of the sterile field and near the nurse so that stretching over the equipment is not necessary. The tips of equipment expected to touch the swabs should not touch each other.

Figure 11.1 Sterile field layout. The sterile field is laid out so that the risk of contamination is reduced. The gallipots or receivers are placed nearest the patient so that fluid is less likely to be dripped across the sterile field. Micro-organisms travel from unsterile environments through wet material; the aim, therefore, is to keep the sterile field dry (Perry and Potter 1998).

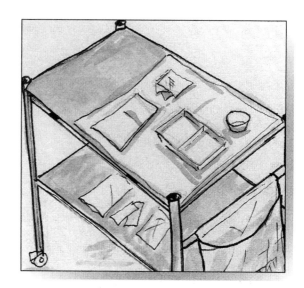

Clean swabs and dressings can be placed in an area of the sterile field so that they are well away from the other equipment, but are ready for use.

Reduction of airborne organisms

It is estimated that approximately 10 per cent of hospital infections result from airborne micro-organisms (Rowley 2001). Contamination of wounds or equipment by airborne bacteria has not been consistently proven, but micro-organisms may be stirred up from movement of personnel, bedmaking and drawing curtains (Briggs et al. 1996). The greatest source of infection may be the general cleanliness of the environment. Ideally, a designated area that has pressure-controlled air exchanges, such as a ward treatment room, should be used. Accepted practice aims to reduce the amount of air movement in the area during an aseptic procedure (AORN 1996). Sensible precautions therefore usually take the following forms:

- closure of curtains and arrangement of bedclothes before sterile equipment is taken into the bed area
- windows and doors are shut, and movement in and out of the curtains is kept to the minimum
- ward cleaning is completed 30 minutes before and avoided during the procedure.

Clean environment and patient

The standards of cleanliness in hospitals have been much criticized recently, and the government response has been to publish standard principles for hospital environmental hygiene (Department of Health 2001a). These encompass a wide range of routine activities that contribute to the prevention of hospital-acquired infection, and include guidelines on cleanliness of the environment and standards of clinical practice.

The areas that are used for aseptic procedures should be physically clean, with appropriate disposal of all clinical waste. Plan procedures to attend to clean wounds before infected ones (AORN 1996). The degree of cleanliness is more difficult to control in a patient's home, but the nurse should ensure that the risks of contamination from the environment are kept to a minimum. For example, a patient's pet may need to be excluded from the room during the aseptic procedure to reduce contamination.

Hands should be decontaminated immediately before and after each and every episode of direct patient care (see Chapter 3). The use of protective clothing such as gloves and aprons should also follow infection control guidelines. For aseptic procedures, sterile gloves are worn.

Additional precautions include the following:

- When using an examination couch for procedures, a protective disposable paper sheet should be changed between patients, and the couch should be disinfected daily or when visibly contaminated.
- The bedclothes should be protected with a waterproof sheet or absorbent pad to prevent irrigation fluid seeping through bedclothes and contaminating the mattress (Perry and Potter 1998).

Self-contamination

A patient's own flora from the gastro-intestinal tract, skin or respiratory tract may infect a wound or an intravenous or urinary catheter (Ayliffe et al. 1999). Helping a patient maintain personal cleanliness, such as using an antiseptic skin preparation before a procedure, offering handwashing facilities after toileting, and using separate wash cloths for face and perineal areas will reduce this risk.

Handwashing

Effective handwashing, following infection control guidelines (see Chapter 3), will reduce contamination risks between patients, and is the single most important activity to prevent transmission of infection. There is confusion as to how often and at what junctures handwashing should occur during an aseptic procedure, which results in ritualistic and/or contradictory practices (Bree-Williams and Waterman 1996).

If considering the principles of asepsis, the following can be used as a guide to handwashing during an aseptic procedure:

- Prior to preparing equipment and patient, a social handwash (see Chapter 3) can be used to remove all transient micro-organisms and physical dirt. A full disinfection handwash is not necessary until everything is ready to begin the sterile procedure, as the hands will be touching a number of objects ranging from equipment to patient bedclothes during preparation.

- Opening additional packs and fluids to add to the sterile field will bring the hands into contact with dry, dust-free equipment that carries a low level of pathogenic activity (Hollingworth and Kingston 1998), and therefore has a low risk of contamination. Provided the sterile products are not touched, physically clean hands may open the packs.

- Whether using the sterile bag technique or forceps to lay out the sterile field and remove a soiled dressing, hand cleansing, either by washing or alcohol disinfection, may be undertaken after removal of the dressing, as that is the most likely time of contamination prior to commencing the procedure. Using a sterile bag to lay out the sterile field has not brought the hands into contact with anything unsterile that will then contact the patient directly until the wound is exposed.

- A disinfection handwash should be undertaken before application of sterile gloves, which may then be worn to proceed.

- If the hands have become contaminated at any stage during the procedure, they can be disinfected using an alcohol hand rub, using two applications and rubbing as for handwashing, provided they are physically clean. This will not be appropriate if there is physical dirt as the alcohol will not be effective (Department of Health 2001a).

NURSING PROBLEM 11.1

Patient history: Mrs Cameron is a 64-year-old lady who has had an emergency laparotomy for abdominal pain.

Problem: Mrs Cameron requires a post-operative wound dressing.

Goal: Mrs Cameron's wound will heal successfully with no infection.

Intervention: aseptic dressing technique

Equipment

- A dressing pack containing a dressing towel, gauze swabs, and gallipot for irrigation fluid; possibly also including waste disposal bag, forceps, or sterile gloves.
- Cleaning lotion, such as sterile saline, or prepacked irrigation device.
- 10 ml syringe.
- Receiver/jug containing hand-hot water for warming the irrigation solution.
- Sterile disposable gloves.
- Alcohol hand rub.
- Tape.
- Additional dressings and wound care products as prescribed.
- Clean scissors for cutting tape. Scissors that have been washed in detergent and dried, or cleaned with an alcohol swab, may be used to cut tape. If scissors are required to cut dressings, for example, to make a keyhole shape, then they should be sterile.
- Receiver to collect irrigation fluid if required.
- Waterproof protection for the bed if irrigation is required.

Procedure

- Clarify the procedure required from the nursing notes. Check for special instructions, such as the type of dressing to be used, to enable appropriate equipment to be selected. Some wounds may require a regular photographic record to monitor progress, or a wound map may be required.

- Identify the Mrs Cameron by name and gain her verbal consent for the procedure. This ensures her cooperation. Ensure you maintain her privacy and dignity by drawing the curtains while checking the current dressing to find out whether additional equipment, such as extra gauze, will be required. Check the type of tape securing the dressing and observe for any discomfort or inflammation in the area so that an appropriate hypoallergenic fixture is used.

- Assess Mrs Cameron's pain score. If necessary, administer analgesia prior to the dressing. This will allow the analgesia to begin to work by the time the dressing is ready to commence.

- Offer toilet facilities to ensure comfort during the procedure.

- Position Mrs Cameron comfortably, maintaining her dignity, privacy and warmth at all times. If there is likely to be only a short interval before you return to commence the procedure, close the curtains and position the bedcovers for easy access to the site. If the wait is likely to be more than 5–10 minutes, don't close the curtains until the equipment is ready: a long wait behind curtains can be worrying for some patients, and may increase anxiety.

- Ensure that all your jewellery is removed other than a wedding ring. This ensures that hands can be washed effectively. Nails should be short and clean.

- Ensure hair is tidy and clipped out of the face. Hair can harbour micro-organisms, and touching it during an aseptic procedure will contaminate the hands.

- Wash hands with a socially clean wash. A clean, disposable apron should be worn for each procedure.

- Ensure the trolley is physically clean and has been washed with detergent that day.

- Gather required equipment (see above), and check for sterile seals, integrity of packaging and expiry dates. Place on the bottom of the trolley and transport to the patient.

- The curtains should be closed and Mrs Cameron positioned comfortably. If the bed height or couch can be raised, position it at about waist level, which should be a comfortable height for working at in order to reduce back strain.

- Ensure a good light source so that you can see the area to be worked on clearly.

TIP!
If undertaking an aseptic procedure in the patient's home, use a designated, hard, flat surface on which to place your equipment. It can be wiped clean of dust and positioned adjacent to the patient.

Preparation of a sterile field

This procedure can be followed for all aseptic procedures.

- Position the trolley beside Mrs Cameron, and on the side nearest to the area that is to be worked on, preferably so that her face and expression can be observed during the procedure. You can see whether she is suffering any undue distress during the procedure that could be relieved by explanation and reassurance.
- Open the dressing pack and slide the inner pack onto the top of the trolley. If there are forceps, an instrument bag, or a waste bag tucked into the packaging, take out and put on one side of the trolley.
- Wash hands with a disinfection wash and dry thoroughly.
- Consider the outer inch of the sterile towel as unsterile; hold about an inch of the corners of the pack. Start with the corner furthest from you, open outwards and straighten out, then the sides, and then the corner nearest you, until the sheet is stretched out flat (Figure 11.2.1). This prevents contamination of the sterile field. Adjust the sterile field so that it is square.

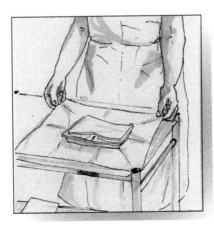

Figure 11.2.1
Straighten out
sterile towel.

● Lay out the area as in Figure 11.1 (page 278) by placing your hand inside the disposal bag (Figure 11.2.2), and positioning the sterile equipment. Forceps may be used to arrange the sterile field instead of the waste bag, and then placed carefully to one side on the sterile field so that the rest of the equipment is not contaminated.

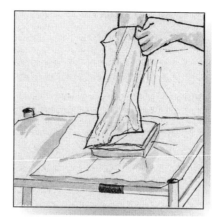

Figure 11.2.2
Using disposal
bag to position
equipment.

● Additional equipment is added by peeling the outer packaging apart, removing by sterile forceps, and positioning on the sterile field. If forceps are not used, the contents can be allowed to slip out of the packaging, taking care not to touch the sterile field with the outer pack, and not to allow equipment to roll off the edge (Figure 11.2.3).

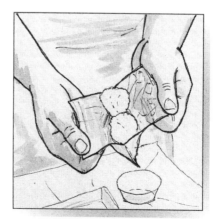

Figure 11.2.3
Opening
additional
equipment.

- Lotions should be poured carefully from the side. If using a multi-dose bottle the label should turn away from the pouring side to prevent drips (Figure 11.2.4). If forceps are being used, a gallipot may be picked up and held to one side, away from the sterile field, while the lotion is poured in.

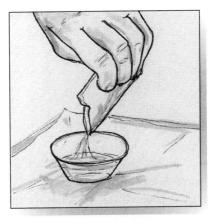

Figure 11.2.4
Pouring lotions from a sachet.

TIP! If assisting at an aseptic procedure, the label of the lotion should be checked with the other health care professional so that you are both satisfied that the correct substance is being used.

- Open sterile gloves and place on top of the sterile field (see Figure 11.4 below).
- Loosen tape on the dressing.
- Place your hand inside the sterile bag, and remove the old dressing, discreetly observing the discharge on the wound dressing on removal.
- Gather all dressing material up into the bag (Figure 11.3), turn inside out and secure on the trolley below the level of the sterile field, but on the same side as the dressing to allow easy disposal of waste during the procedure.
- If forceps are used to remove the old dressing, they are then returned for resterilizing if metal, or discarded.
- Clean hands either by a disinfection wash or alcohol rub. Dry thoroughly.
- Put on sterile gloves.

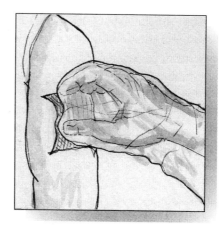

Figure 11.3
Removing old
dressing.

● Assess the wound: observe the wound and surrounding area for inflammation, swelling, or discharge. Do not allow the wound to remain uncovered for too long as the temperature will drop and interrupt healing.

● If the *skin around* the wound needs cleaning, it can be swabbed by gauze swabs slightly moistened with sterile saline. The *wound should not* be swabbed with gauze or cotton wool as fibres may enter the wound bed, and cause a foreign body reaction (Briggs et al. 1996).

● To *clean around* a wound, wipe from top to bottom, or from clean area to dirty if that is more obvious, using one wipe for each swab.

● If the wound needs cleaning, fill a 10 ml syringe with sterile saline, or use a prepacked irrigation device.

● Placing the sterile receiver below the wound to catch the flow, irrigate the wound with the syringe, ensuring that it does not touch the wound. The pressure at which to irrigate has not been confirmed (Oliver 1997) but should be sufficient to flush away surface debris without causing trauma. If a small irrigation only is required, fluid may be collected by holding a gauze swab below the wound.

● Dry the *surrounding skin* with dry gauze, working from top to bottom or clean to dirty as before.

● Position the prescribed dressing and secure. Tape pieces should be cut individually and applied, but the tape should not be carried to the wound as it may become contaminated.

- On completion, fold up sterile field, remove apron and gloves, and deposit all in waste bag. All waste should be wrapped before leaving the area (to reduce transmission of infection outside the treatment area) and disposed of as clinical waste (Xavier 1999).
- Before leaving Mrs Cameron, position her comfortably, ensuring all that she requires is within reach.
- Equipment for resterilizing should be placed on the top of the trolley and returned to the dirty utility room; if it contains body secretions, it should be rinsed before being returned to CSSD.

TIP! Where sharps have been used as part of an aseptic procedure, it is the responsibility of the practitioner using the sharp (e.g. needle or stitch-cutter) to ensure its safe disposal in an appropriate container (see Chapter 3).

- After waste disposal, wash hands. Document activity and observations.

Evaluation

Mrs Cameron's wound heals by first intention (i.e. without evidence of infection).

Putting on sterile gloves

TIP! Choose the correct size to ensure a comfortable fit and ease of manipulation, and to reduce potential breaks in the gloves.

- Open outer packaging and allow contents to slip onto flat surface (Figure 11.4.1).
- Following disinfection handwash and thorough drying, open inner packaging
- Using your non-dominant hand, pick up the opposite glove (Figure 11.4.2) by grasping the exposed inside of the cuff (i.e. left hand picks up right glove, or right hand picks up left glove).
- Pull the glove onto your dominant hand, keeping your thumb folded across your palm to avoid touching the sterile outside of the glove (Figure 11.4.3). Hold the cuff on the inside until your fingers have entered the appropriate glove fingers and wriggled into place, then allow the cuff to unroll a little (Figure 11.4.4).

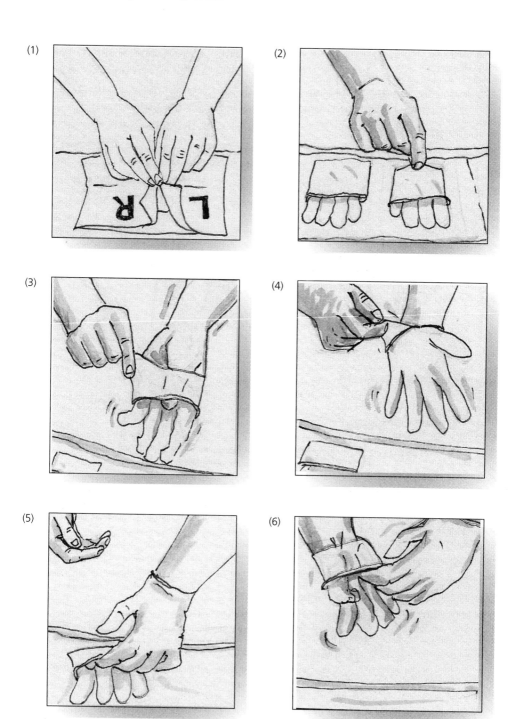

Figure 11.4.1–6 Donning sterile gloves.

- Using your gloved hand, slip your finger under the cuff of the other glove to pick it up (Figure 11.4.5). Slide your non-dominant hand into the glove, keeping the thumb tucked in until it is fully covered. The dominant hand can release the glove when placed correctly. Be careful not to contaminate the fingers when straightening the cuffs of either hand (Figure 11.4.6).
- The gloves can be adjusted to fit comfortably by interlacing the fingers of both hands and smoothing the material. The gloves will remain sterile so long as they only touch sterile materials.

TIP! Wearing sterile gloves can give you a false sense of security that may lead to contamination of key parts when handling equipment, so be vigilant and maintain ANTT.

NURSING PROBLEM 11.2

Problem: Mrs Cameron has a wound drain in situ that requires shortening after 24 hours, and removal after 48 hours.
Goal: Mrs Cameron's wound drain is shortened and removed safely and without discomfort.

Wound drains

Wound drains are designed to aid drainage of fluids such as pus, blood, or exudate from a body cavity. Accumulation of such fluids increases the risk of infection and may delay wound healing, but the presence of a drain may act as a conduit for micro-organisms (Briggs 1997). Manley and Bellman (2000) suggest that drains should be removed in the following circumstances:

- when the drain no longer fulfils its function, and drainage is minimal or nil
- suction drains should be removed when there is less than 50 ml drainage in 24 hours
- when an abscess cavity is confirmed by radiology as being closed
- when there is a risk of complications occurring due to the location and length of time in situ.

The decision to remove a drain should be confirmed by a qualified nurse or medical practitioner.

The many different types of drains are well documented elsewhere, but the principles of shortening and removal are outlined in the following procedure.

TIP! When shortening or removing a wound drain, ensure that the patient has had some effective pain relief. This will help them relax and cooperate, and relieve discomfort following removal.

Intervention: shortening a wound drain

Equipment

As for aseptic dressing technique (see page 281) but also:

- Sterile stitch cutter.
- Sterile forceps.
- Sterile safety pin.

Procedure

- Prepare for procedure following the steps described for the aseptic dressing technique (page 281) up to the stage of wound assessment.
- Expose the wound drain site, and clean the surrounding skin if necessary.
- A drain may be repositioned by removing the suture that is securing it in position. Identify the suture holding it in situ and, lifting it with the sterile forceps, cut the suture under the knot, next to the skin, and gently remove the suture.
- Withdraw the drain the prescribed distance (usually 2–3 cm), warning the patient that she may experience a pulling sensation. Take a gauze pad and with the non-dominant hand hold it at the drain site, applying slight counter-pressure to the skin around the wound. With the other hand, gently pull the drain. If resistance is felt or the patient complains of discomfort, pause and slow down. Encourage the patient to take deep breaths to help her relax whilst you shorten the drain.

- Insert the sterile safety pin through the drain at the new length to prevent it slipping back into the wound.
- Dry the skin around the wound with gauze swab.
- A keyhole dressing (Figure 11.5) is applied around the drain, and additional gauze placed over the drain and secured.

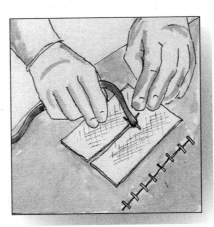

Figure 11.5
Keyhole dressing.

TIP! If there are copious amounts of drainage, a stoma bag may be used rather than a dressing to collect discharge. Aseptic precautions should be adhered to when placing the bag in situ.

- Complete the aseptic procedure as described on page 286.
- Record type and amount of drainage, and the condition of the wound.

Intervention: removing a wound drain

Equipment

As for aseptic dressing technique (see page 281) but also:

- Sterile stitch cutter.
- Sterile forceps.
- Specimen jar if signs of local infection are present.

Procedure

- Prepare for procedure and position the patient following the steps described for the aseptic dressing technique (page 281) up to the stage of wound assessment.
- If the drain is by vacuum, discontinue the vacuum by clamping the drain.
- Expose the wound drain site, and clean the surrounding skin if necessary.
- If a suture is still in situ, identify the suture and, lifting it with the sterile forceps, cut the suture under the knot, next to the skin, and gently remove the suture.
- Warn the patient that she may experience a pulling sensation as you remove the drain.
- Take a gauze pad and with the non-dominant hand hold it at the drain site, applying slight counter-pressure to the skin around the wound. With the other hand gently pull the drain out. If resistance is felt or the patient complains of discomfort, pause and slow down. Encourage the patient to take deep breaths while you remove the drain.
- Discard the drain into the waste bag, taking note of the colour or odour of any discharge. If there are signs of infection, place the drain in a specimen jar to send for microscopy and culture.
- Apply gentle pressure with a gauze swab until any bleeding or drainage from the site has stopped, and then apply a sterile dressing.
- Complete the aseptic procedure as described on page 286.
- Record the type and amount of drainage, and the condition of the wound.

Evaluation

Has Mrs Cameron's wound drain been effective? Are there any signs of fluid collecting internally – i.e. evidence of haematoma (bruising), swelling, heat or pain? Is the wound healing as expected?

NURSING PROBLEM 11.3

Problem: Mrs Cameron requires removal of sutures.

Goal: Mrs Cameron's sutures will be removed from a healed and intact wound site at post-operative day x.

Sutures

Wound closures such as sutures and staples are used to hold wound edges together in apposition to promote healing without infection. Before removal, it is necessary to determine the type of wound closure so that the correct removal technique is used and also the appropriate equipment, e.g. a staple or clip remover, scissors or stitch cutter. This should be written in the nursing notes and surgical record. The timing of removal depends on the position of the wound. For example, facial sutures may be removed within 3 to 5 days, but abdominal retention sutures may remain until 14–21 days post-operatively (Torrance and Serginson 1997).

The main principle to remember when removing sutures is that any part of the suture that has been exposed on the skin surface should not travel under the skin as it is removed, since it is likely to take surface micro-organisms into the wound area. This means that cutting the suture must be carefully planned (Figure 11.6). Never cut both ends of a visible suture or you will not be able to extract the suture from below the skin surface.

TIP! **Clips or staples are removed using a specific clip or staple remover, which may differ depending on the type of skin closure used. Check by reading the patient's notes before you start the procedure that you have the correct instrument available.**

Intervention: removal of skin closures (sutures/staples)

Equipment

Equipment as for aseptic technique but also:

● Sterile stitch cutter or appropriate closure remover.
● Sterile forceps.

Procedure

● Prepare for procedure and position the patient following the steps described for the aseptic dressing technique (page 281) up to the stage of wound assessment.
● Inspect the wound for evidence of healing. If there are signs of inflammation or discharge consult with the nurse in charge to determine the appropriate strategy for removal, and take a wound swab for microscopy and culture before proceeding.
● Lift the suture knot with forceps, cut the suture under the knot nearest the skin and lift upwards, supporting the skin with the non-dominant hand as the movement pulls on the wound (Figure 11.6). Discard. For long or deep wounds alternate sutures are removed first to ascertain whether the wound has healed consistently throughout.

TIP! **Some suture holes may discharge exudate or pus, indicating localized infection which may resolve when the sutures have been removed. These individual sutures should be removed and an adhesive skin closure used to maintain apposition of the wound. More generalized swelling and redness may indicate a deeper wound infection and removal of skin closure may result in part of the wound opening (wound dehiscence) and discharge of exudate. Advice from an experienced nurse should be sought before skin closures on such a wound are removed.**

● If a staple or clip remover is used, it usually operates by squeezing the centre of the clip so that the edges are lifted out of the skin (Figure 11.7). The patient may feel some slight 'tweaking' or 'pulling' of the wound site during the procedure. Support the skin on either side of the wound with the non-dominant hand during the procedure.

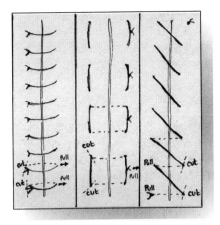

Figure 11.6
Cutting sutures.

Figure 11.7
Using a clip
remover.

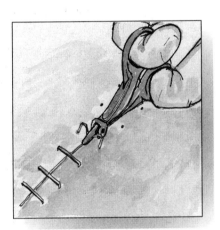

- If the wound is healing well and skin edges are healed the wound closures may be removed. Some patients prefer a dry dressing (as a comfort and protection measure) over the wound for a few days until the scab has fallen off, depending on the location of the wound.
- Complete the procedure as described before for the aseptic dressing technique (page 286).

Evaluation

Have Mrs Cameron's wound closures been removed safely and completely and is her wound healing well?

NURSING PROBLEM 11.4

Problem: Mrs Cameron has evidence of a wound infection.

Goal: To detect the type of infection to enable appropriate treatment.

Intervention: taking a wound swab

Swabs can be taken from various sites, and sent for culture. If infection is suspected a swab should be taken before antibiotic treatment is commenced. If there is likely to be a delay between collection and arrival at the laboratory, the swab may be transported in a special culture medium to maintain moisture and viability. Check local practices when collecting and transporting wound swabs.

Collection of a wound swab usually occurs at the beginning of an aseptic dressing procedure, before any treatment has commenced.

Equipment

- Sterile wound swab and request form.
- Culture medium if required.

Procedure

- Prepare for procedure following the steps described for the aseptic dressing technique (page 281) up to the stage of wound assessment.
- Explain to Mrs Cameron why and how you are going to take a swab and how it will help her recovery.
- Remove wound dressing. If infection is suspected, the wound and the surrounding skin may be inflamed, hot and painful, with a purulent exudate from the wound itself.
- Open the wound swab and wipe some exudate onto the swab (Figure 11.8). Take care not to touch the surrounding skin or to contaminate the swab or yourself. Provided a non-touch technique is maintained, wearing gloves is not necessary (ANTT).
- Replace the swab carefully into the transport container or transport medium, depending on local policy requirements, without touching the sides.

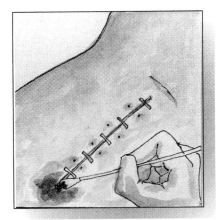

Figure 11.8
Taking a wound
swab.

- Label the specimen with the following information: the patient's name; identity number; the site from where it was collected; and the date and time of collection.
- Ensure that the accompanying request form is completed with the following information: the patient's name and number; diagnosis, e.g. emergency laparotomy; type of specimen, e.g. wound exudate from lower abdominal incision; relevant history, e.g. abdominal surgery 7 days ago; relevant drugs such as antibiotics; and requesting doctor's name and signature and consultant.
- Wash hands before progressing further with care.

Evaluation

Mrs Cameron's wound swab will provide sufficient bacterial growth when cultured to identify the type of infection to enable appropriate treatment to be prescribed.

Assisting at an aseptic procedure

When preparing for an aseptic procedure and you are asked to prepare equipment for it, look up the specific requirements in the local clinical guidelines to ensure that you have considered the stages of the procedure and have got equipment for each stage; for example:

- something to clean the patient's skin, e.g. antiseptic lotion
- local anaesthetic to reduce pain; needles and syringe or applicator to administer it

- specific aseptic pack, e.g. catheterization or lumbar puncture
- gloves: ask for specific size required, plus a spare in case of a tear
- wound closures, e.g. sutures or specific dressing
- tape
- hand disinfection lotion
- specimen container
- small sharps container for easy disposal of scalpels or needles.

When assisting during the procedure:

- Position and prepare the patient, and support her. You may be asked to help her maintain a particular position or hold her hand during the procedure.
- If you are required to open the sterile field, ensure that you have washed your hands with a disinfection wash between positioning the patient and assisting with the equipment.
- Open additional packs as required, such as gloves, needles and syringes. The pack should be opened by peeling back the packaging, and the contents carefully slipped onto the sterile field (Figure 11.4), or taken from you by the operator. Be careful not to drop contents from a height as they may slip off the sterile field and onto the floor.
- When tidying up afterwards first identify any sharps and make safe by disposal into the sharps box or by putting in an obvious location, such as a gallipot, for disposal immediately on leaving the location, before other equipment is discarded.
- Ensure the patient is left clean, comfortable and with the call bell within reach.
- If any observations are to be maintained following the procedure, ensure you start and continue them and record on appropriate record sheet.
- Ensure any specimens taken during the procedure are labelled and packaged appropriately and have appropriate request forms completed and signed to accompany the specimen.

Male and female catheterization

The placement of an indwelling urinary catheter is an aseptic procedure as it involves breaching the body's natural defences by inserting a catheter through the urinary meatus. There is consistent evidence that a significant number of hospital-acquired infections are related to urinary catheterization (Department of Health 2001b), and therefore the decision to use an indwelling urinary catheter should be considered carefully. Infections are reduced when a closed drainage system is used and when catheters are left in situ for as short a time as possible. Because of the high level of associated infection with urinary catheterization, it should not be the first line of treatment when treating urinary incontinence (Simpson 2001).

Urinary catheterization is undertaken in the following cases (Simpson 2001):

- to relieve bladder distension resulting from acute urine retention or urinary tract obstruction
- to drain an acute or chronic (neurogenic) paralysed bladder
- to detect incomplete bladder emptying and measure residual urine
- to monitor urine output in serious illness
- for pre-/post-operative drainage, particularly during pelvic and abdominal surgery
- to investigate urodynamics
- to instil drugs into the bladder
- to manage catheter patency
- to manage intractable urinary incontinence.

The type of catheter used depends on patient needs and expected duration of catheterization. Short-term catheterization is considered to be between 14 and 28 days, and long-term up to three months or more. Teflon-coated latex catheters are adequate for short-term use, but uncoated latex catheters are avoided to prevent complications developing, such as latex allergy, infection and encrustation. For long-term use, silicone catheters, silicone elastomer-coated or hydrogel-coated latex catheters are acceptable (Parker 1999).

Ideally, the smallest size that allows free flow of urine is selected, with a 10 ml balloon, as this minimizes urethral trauma, mucosal irritation and residual urine in the bladder which predispose to catheter associated infection (Department of Health 2001b). The average size for women is 12–14 FG, and for men 14–16 FG. Patients with specific urological problems may require large catheters; it is therefore essential to check the patient's notes to check for specific orders. The Department of Health (2001b) recommendations note that urethral damage and subsequent pain and discomfort, particularly in male patients, is lessened if an experienced practitioner inserts the catheter.

This reinforces the importance of ensuring you are adequately supervised when learning clinical skills.

It is only recently that female nurses have begun to catheterize male patients. Milligan (1999) suggests that this is less likely to be related to the difficulty of the procedure than to the psychosexual connotations that are linked with male genitalia, masculine body image and sexuality, and suggests that catheterization may be perceived as an invasion of an individual's sexuality. Experience suggests that some women may find their sexual beliefs and gender attitudes challenged by a male nurse catheterizing them. Space precludes full discussion of these issues within this chapter but when caring for a patient with a catheter, you need to be sensitive to these issues and be concerned to support a patient's dignity, privacy and perception of body image and sexual identity during catheterization and catheter care.

NURSING PROBLEM 11.5

Patient history: Mrs Jaffrey has been admitted in a semi-comatose state and appears dehydrated. She requires accurate fluid output measurement.

Problem: Mrs Jaffrey requires a urinary catheter to monitor urine output. The presence of a urinary catheter predisposes to a urine infection.

Goal: Mrs Jaffrey output will return to a urine output of at least 1.5 litres per 24 hrs.

Patient history: Mr Gregg is a 63-year-old gentleman who has not been able to pass urine for 24 hours. He is in a lot of discomfort due to acute retention of urine.

Problem: Mr Gregg has acute retention of urine and requires urinary catheterization.

Goal: Mr Gregg's urine retention will be relieved and normal flow restored.

Intervention: female and male catheterization

Equipment

- Catheter pack, containing gallipot, receiver, dressing towels and/or waterproof sheet, gauze swabs, specimen pot.
- Lubricant/anaesthetic gel depending on local policy.
- Cleansing agent such as 0.9% saline solution.
- 10 ml syringe and needle.
- 10 ml ampoule water for injection.
- Two pairs of sterile gloves, appropriate size.
- Two catheters of appropriate size and type according to local policy and patient's requirements (e.g. 12 or 14 FG for female short-term catheterization, 14 or 16 FG for male).
- Urine drainage bag and hanger.
- Disposable waterproof pad, such as an incontinence pad.
- Alcohol handrub.

Procedure

- Prepare the patient as for an aseptic procedure, explaining the procedure and maintaining privacy, dignity and warmth. Gain the patient's verbal consent if possible. Ideally, catheterization should take place after general personal hygiene has been attended to, as studies indicate that routine meatal hygiene using soap and water is less abrasive and as effective as any other preparation using antiseptic or microbial substances (Department of Health 2001b).
- Wash hands using a social wash and gather equipment onto a clean, dry trolley.
- Transport the trolley to the patient and position it with the nurse's dominant hand next to the patient. Close the curtains and position the patient.
- Female: Mrs Jaffrey may lie supine or at 45°, with her knees bent and thighs apart, exposing the genital area. Pillows may be used outside the knees to support legs in this position to maintain patient comfort. An elderly patient may find this a difficult or painful position to maintain, and so may prefer to lie on her side, with the upper leg flexed at the hip and knee joints and supported by a pillow.

- Male: Mr Gregg may lie supine or at 45°, with the genital area exposed.
- Fold bedclothes away from genital area and place disposable waterproof pad under the buttocks.
- Position a good light source such that the genital area is well illuminated.

TIP! **Positioning a light source before commencing an aseptic procedure is worth spending some time and effort on. Remember that your head may obscure it while you are working, and so it should be placed where the site can be clearly seen but where your head will not block the light, or hit it if you change position.**

- Open the catheter pack and place inner contents onto the trolley surface.
- Wash hands with a disinfection wash and dry thoroughly.
- Lay out the sterile field, ensuring that the gallipot is placed nearest to the patient to prevent fluid from contaminating the sterile area (Figure 11.2).
- Empty saline sachet into the gallipot.
- Open catheter and place in its inner wrapping in the receiver.
- Draw up the 10 ml water (or required amount of fluid to fill the balloon) into the syringe and place to one side.
- For female patients, squeeze about 3 cm of lubricant/anaesthetic gel onto a piece of gauze and place to one side.
- Prepare the lubricant/anaesthetic gel according to manufacturer's instructions.

TIP! **Lignocaine 2% gel should not cause any side effects when applied topically, but it should be prescribed on the patient's prescription sheet. Check that it is compatible with any other medication that the patient receives.**

- Open the catheter drainage bag and, ensuring the connecting end remains covered, attach the bag to the bed on a hanger, and place the connection within reach.
- Open *two* pairs of sterile gloves on the sterile field.
- Place sterile dressing towels between and over the patient's thighs.

- Disinfect hands either by washing or hand rub.
- Put on *two* pairs of sterile gloves.
- Female (F): take a gauze swab in the non-dominant hand and using your thumb, middle and index fingers separate the labia to provide a clear view of the urinary meatus (Figure 11.9). The swab is used to maintain separation of the labia whilst the area is prepared.
- F: use a gauze swab and saline solution to clean the inner labia, using a downward wipe towards the anus and using a fresh swab for each wipe, and discarding each swab after use into the clinical waste bag. Clean each side and then the meatus.
- F: if your local policy requires it, instil 10 ml anaesthetic gel into the urinary meatus (Addison 2000). A wait of at least 3–5 minutes is necessary before it is effective. Research has not confirmed the efficacy of lignocaine gel for female catheterization but it is thought to minimize urethral trauma and reduce infection if used (Department of Health 2001b).
- F: remove top pair of gloves and discard.
- F: take the receiver with the catheter in, and place between Mrs Jaffrey's thighs. Remove the top of the catheter wrapper. Ensure the catheter is not contaminated by touching anything non-sterile in the immediate vicinity.
- F: lubricate the tip of the catheter with gel on the gauze.
- F: remove gauze from labia and discard, keeping the labia open with the hand. Insert the catheter gently, following a natural

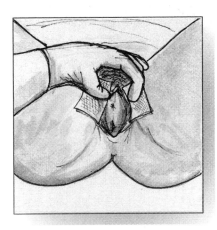

Figure 11.9
Separation of the female labia.

pathway – slightly upwards and backwards. It may help if the patient bears down or coughs. If there is any resistance, stop. Check the position of the catheter as it may slip into the vagina.

TIP! If the catheter inadvertently goes into the vagina, leave it there as a marker, and start afresh with a new catheter. Once the catheter is in position, remove the first catheter.

- F: advance the catheter for about 10–12 cm in total until urine flows into the receiver. Advance the catheter a further 5 mm to ensure it has fully entered the bladder.
- Inflate the balloon with the pre-filled syringe of water, taking note of how many millilitres are used.
- Continue as described below (page 305) for the final stages of the procedure.
- Male (M): hold the penis by the non-dominant hand and lift to an angle of 60–90° to allow effective cleansing and local anaesthetic to take effect.
- M: clean the glans penis with a moistened gauze swab, using a locally specified cleaning agent, such as sterile saline solution. In uncircumcised patients, retract the foreskin and clean the urinary meatus. Use a circulatory motion, starting at the centre and working outwards.

WARNING!

If you have difficulty identifying the urethral meatus due to phimosis (prepuce cannot be drawn back over the glans penis) do not continue, but summon expert assistance.

- M: instil 20 ml anaesthetic gel (Addison 2000) into the urinary meatus using the applicator provided. To prevent gel from being expelled from the urethra, hold the tip of the glans penis firmly with the non-dominant hand, and wipe the underside of the penis downwards to allow the anaesthetic to take effect along the urethra. While the anaesthetic gel is taking effect, place penis on a piece of gauze.
- M: remove the top pair of gloves.

- M: take the receiver with the catheter in and place between Mr Gregg's thighs.
- M: tear the catheter wrapper along the perforations and, holding the penis in the non-dominant hand at an angle of 60–90°, insert the catheter into the urethra for 15–25 cm until urine begins to flow. Draw back the wrapper from the catheter as it advances. If resistance is met, straighten the penis a little more and ask the patient to cough or bear down to enable the catheter to pass through the internal sphincter. Medical assistance should be sought if there is pain or evidence of trauma such as bleeding.
- M: once urine has started to flow, advance the catheter 5 cm more to ensure it is fully in the bladder.
- M: inflate the balloon with the required amount of water, taking note of how much is used. If there is any pain or discomfort when doing this, stop the proceedings as it may indicate the catheter is not fully in the bladder.
- M: replace the foreskin, and wipe away any excess anaesthetic gel.

TIP! **If a patient is catheterized for acute retention of urine, the sudden release of a large amount of fluid from the bladder may precipitate hypovolaemic shock. Careful observation of the amount and speed of urine drained may detect an early change in the patient's condition as well as pulse and blood pressure recordings. Local policy may require a regime of clamping the catheter at intervals to prevent too rapid a reduction in bladder volume.**

- The final stages in this procedure apply for both males and females.
- Attach the catheter to the drainage bag, and ensure the bag is hung below the level of the bladder at all times to prevent backflow of urine. Tape the drainage bag to the thigh to prevent it pulling on the urethra.
- A specimen of urine may be taken from the sterile receiver or catheter wrapper and sent for microscopy and culture if required.
- Place the equipment onto the top of the trolley and position the patient comfortably, ensuring that all immediate needs are within reach.
- Place all waste into bag, including discarded apron and gloves. Leave the bed area.
- Discard waste and wash hands.

- Record your actions, including: reason for catheterization; date and time of insertion; type/size of catheter used; batch number, manufacturer, and expiry date; amount of water used to inflate the balloon; amount of urine drained at catheterization; and when catheterization should be reviewed (adapted from Simpson 2001).

TIP! **Patients who are catheterized should have an intake of at least 2–3 litres of fluid daily to keep urine dilute and reduce infection risks. Plan with patients to increase fluid intake daily and consider ways of increasing 'hidden fluids' within their usual dietary habits (Simpson 2001; see also Chapter 7 in this book).**

Evaluation

Is the urine flowing freely? What is the colour, concentration, and amount? Can you smell any evidence of infection?

For further catheter care, see Chapter 10.

Further reading

AORN (1996) Recommended practices for maintaining a sterile field. AORN Journal 64(5): 817–21.

Ayliffe GAJ, Babb JR, Taylor LJ (1999) Hospital-Acquired Infection: Principles and Prevention, 3rd edn. Oxford: Butterworth-Heinemann.

Bree-Williams FJ, Waterman H (1996) An examination of nurses' practices when performing aseptic technique for wound dressings. Journal of Advanced Nursing 23(1): 48–54.

Briggs M, Wilson S, Fuller A (1996) The principles of aseptic technique in wound care. Professional Nurse 11(12): 805–12.

Manley K, Bellman L (eds) (2000) Surgical Nursing: Advancing Practice. Edinburgh: Churchill Livingstone.

CHAPTER 12

Principles of pre- and post-operative care

Aims and learning outcomes

This chapter outlines the key principles of preparation of a patient for a surgical or investigative procedure requiring sedation or anaesthesia, and summarizes the post-operative care required for a safe recovery. By the end of the chapter, you will be able to:

- undertake safe physical preparation of a patient to prevent complications arising from an anaesthetic or surgical intervention
- be aware of some key psychological factors to be addressed prior to surgery
- receive a patient following recovery from anaesthesia and continue their immediate post-operative care, providing safe recovery from surgical intervention
- identify the nursing interventions required to prevent post-operative complications.

Introduction

Admission for surgery can be planned or as an emergency. Planned surgery means that the patient has been waiting on a list, possibly for some time. The anticipated outcome of the surgery is expected to be good as the surgery is likely to relieve unpleasant or uncomfortable symptoms, or determine their cause. There will have been an opportunity for the patient to make psychological preparations and to begin to adjust to the probable outcome, and therefore he or she may be eager to get on with the process. Health care staff will have the opportunity to prepare the patient to be in the best condition for surgery, thus reducing potential problems. Emergency surgery does not allow the patient to make these preliminary adjustments, and the patient may be feeling so ill that they cannot anticipate what the outcome may be, so will have to adjust to the situation after surgery.

Whatever route patients follow for surgery, the principles for safe preparation and recovery are the same. Time is the major limitation, since patients who attend for planned day surgery have less opportunity to get to know the staff caring for them, and emergency admissions will not have had the opportunity to be in optimal health. The following care plans focus on preparing a patient for a planned surgical intervention, identifing ideal practice and drawing on several of the procedures detailed in previous chapters.

Pre-admission clinic

A visit to a pre-admission clinic about 10 to 14 days before an operation provides the opportunity to undertake a thorough pre-operative assessment prior to admission (Torrance and Serginson 1997). These clinics reduce unnecessary time in hospital waiting for surgery and allow familiarization with the forthcoming procedure so reducing anxiety and preparing for speedy recovery.

Torrance and Serginson (1997) summarize the aim of pre-admission clinics as being to:

- minimize cancellations and maximize the use of beds and theatre space
- improve admission and assessment procedures
- improve discharge planning
- offer full and thorough patient education prior to surgery.

The physical condition of the patient is assessed, and any outstanding investigations – such as a full blood count (FBC), electrocardiogram (ECG), blood cross-matching or lung function tests, or the gathering of other essential medical and social information – are carried out. For an elderly patient or one with complex care needs, this provides the opportunity to assess the degree of support that they will require on discharge from hospital, and begin the process of discharge planning.

The proposed surgical procedure can be discussed and the patient is able to ask questions of the nursing and medical staff. Written information about the operation and expected plan of care may be given to the patient to take away and consider at leisure. This enables the patient to understand treatment options more fully and informed consent can be given.

Any specific preparation prior to surgery can be discussed with the patient such as:

- reducing cigarette intake
- planning weight loss
- stopping the contraceptive pill and taking alternative contraceptive precautions
- skin and hygiene preparation
- bowel preparation.

NURSING PROBLEM 12.1

Patient history: Ms Bailey, a divorced 47-year-old, has been admitted for a total abdominal hysterectomy. She has been a smoker for 30 years, but while waiting for this operation she has managed to reduce her cigarette intake to 5–10 a day.

Problem: Ms Bailey requires pre-operative preparation to prevent complications from a general anaesthetic.

Goal: Ms Bailey will have an uncomplicated recovery from a general anaesthetic.

Intervention: preparation for a general anaesthetic

Record baseline observations: TPR, BP, weight, urinalysis

Vital signs and urinalysis should be taken both to detect any abnormalities (see Chapter 2), and to establish a baseline for post-operative monitoring. Recording weight provides information from which to calculate drug dosages and estimate the patient's nutritional status (see Chapter 9).

Identify pre-existing conditions or allergies

When assessing Ms Bailey it is important to discover if she has experienced any allergic reactions to drugs, skin adhesives, or latex in the past, as these may affect the choice of anaesthetic or treatments during surgery.

Any medications that Ms Bailey may be taking should be recorded, as some will need to be continued throughout the time of hospitalization. Patients may need reminding that oral contraceptives, hormone replacement therapies, and complementary or alternative therapies should be documented as they may affect treatment. For example, some natural remedies can affect blood clotting times.

If Ms Bailey had a chronic condition, such as diabetes mellitus, hypertension or asthma, which required continuous treatment she would need to have her condition and medication recorded so that therapy could be managed appropriately during her admission.

Pre-operative education to promote recovery

Ms Bailey is a smoker of several years' duration and is likely to want to cough post-operatively. She should be taught deep breathing and coughing exercises pre-operatively to prevent a chest infection developing. As she is expected to have an abdominal incision she will find it helpful to learn to support the wound with her hands while she coughs.

Other pre-operative education may include leg exercises to promote circulation in the calves and reduce the potential for post-operative deep vein thrombosis (DVT) and pulmonary embolus (PE). If DVT is a risk, Ms Bailey should be measured and fitted with anti-embolytic stockings to promote good venous return (see Chapter 5).

Post-operative pain relief may be discussed with Ms Bailey, and the option to use patient-controlled analgesia (PCA) may be given. Studies indicate that patients who use PCA post-operatively are discharged from hospital two days earlier than patients who use other methods (Thomas 1995). If Ms Bailey uses a PCA she will be introduced to it pre-operatively and educated in its use.

Fasting (nil by mouth)

Fasting before an anaesthetic reduces the potential for vomiting and aspiration of gastric contents while unconscious which can lead to aspiration pneumonia. If the gastro-intestinal tract is to be operated upon, then fasting and bowel preparation times are likely to be prolonged to allow the bowel to empty and so reduce possible contamination of the abdominal cavity by gastric or faecal contents (Finlay 1996). Local guidelines should be followed for specific bowel preparations.

Studies indicate that clear fluids can be taken up to two hours before operation and food can be consumed up to four hours before an anaesthetic (Seymour 2000). In practice, patients tend to be fasted from a convenient starting time such as 12 midnight, which may mean that there is a long time before they are able to restart eating and drinking. For particularly vulnerable patients like the elderly, this may mean they suffer from hypoglycaemia (low blood sugar), dehydration, ketosis (fat breakdown), confusion and headache. To provide individualized care, fasting times should be tailored to the operating theatre list and the patient's individual needs (Hung 1992).

Explanations should be given to Ms Bailey about the necessity to fast from fluids and food and cigarettes before an anaesthetic. If clear fluids are allowed, then guidelines as to which clear fluids may be taken should be given, as well as specific time limits for drinking which may be dependent on local policies.

Nausea and vomiting

Prolonged or inadequate periods of fasting can contribute to postoperative nausea and vomiting (PONV), and therefore the individual patient, his or her condition, and other predisposing factors should be taken into account (Jolley 2001). These factors include:

- abdominal or gynaecological operations
- tendency to travel-sickness
- migraines
- previous experience of PONV.

Informing Ms Bailey that PONV can be controlled with appropriate medication may alleviate her anxiety about nausea and vomiting, and encourage her to report symptoms early. The anaesthetist can reduce possible PONV by careful choice of anaesthetic and post-operative analgesia (Hutchings 1995).

Removal of nail varnish/make-up/prostheses/ hearing aids

Nail varnish and make-up should be removed so that skin colour and nail beds can be monitored during anaesthesia for any changes in colour that might indicate inadequate perfusion.

Patients who cannot see without their glasses or hear without hearing aids may be permitted to wear these to the anaesthetic room and then hand them over to the accompanying nurse. Hearing aids in particular should be made available immediately post-operatively if the patient is reliant on them to understand his or her surroundings (Dawson 2000). Ensure that it is clearly documented on the patient's notes that a hearing aid is required and state where it has been stored during the operation.

Other prostheses such as hairpieces or wigs or false eyes should be dealt with sensitively. The patient may not want to be seen without them, but may agree to allow the nurse to take them off in the anaesthetic room and return with them to the ward.

Dentures and contact lenses should be removed and stored appropriately in a named container before surgery. A record of any caps, crowns or loose teeth should be made on the patient's notes so damage can be avoided during the induction of the anaesthetic.

Pre-medication

Pre-medications to induce relaxation and reduce anxiety are rarely administered nowadays as their actions prolong the patient's hospital stay, particularly in day cases (Dawson 2000). Additionally, modern anaesthetics are rapid-acting and no longer need a sedative pre-medication, so if pre-medications are given they are more likely to be used to prevent complications from surgery (see 'Nursing problem 12.2'). Emergency cases may have been given analgesia prior to surgery and this may also sedate the patient.

Evaluation

Was Ms Bailey safe for anaesthesia? Did she fast for an optimum period? Can she undertake leg and coughing exercises effectively?

NURSING PROBLEM 12.2

Problem: Ms Bailey needs to be physically prepared to prevent complications arising from surgery.

Goal: Ms Bailey will have an uneventful recovery from surgery.

Intervention: preparation for a surgical procedure

Informed consent

Ms Bailey should have been able to give her consent for surgery, having had appropriate information as to the choices and treatment options available. It is the role of the medical staff to ensure that consent has been given. Nurses may find that a patient wants to discuss some related issues and perhaps clarify the meaning of some medical jargon or technical words (Dawson 2000). Ensure that a suitably qualified nurse is available to discuss the procedure with Ms Bailey.

Skin preparation

Pre-operative skin preparation aims to reduce the presence of dirt and transient micro-organisms, particularly *Staphylococcus aureus*, which has been found to be the most common cause of wound infection (Simmons 1998). Usually a bath or shower using an antiseptic wash on the day is sufficient, but some surgeons require several consecutive days' preparation with antiseptic solutions to reduce skin flora. Studies to confirm the optimum preparation for every operation are as yet inconclusive, although it is known that washing with skin antiseptics prior to surgery does reduce wound infections.

If possible, hair should be washed pre-operatively to reduce the possibility of it acting as a reservoir for infection. Special attention should be paid to cleaning the umbilicus and finger- and toenails, and nail varnish should be removed (Torrance and Serginson 1997).

The debate concerning hair removal before surgery also remains inconclusive. Shaving is known to cause abrasions which are likely to encourage bacterial proliferation. Less infection occurs if the skin is shaved immediately before surgery rather than the previous day (Simmons 1998). Otherwise, clipping is advised for hair that may obscure the surgical field, but the clippers should be well maintained and sterilized between use on patients (Torrance and Serginson 1997). Depilatory (hair-removing) cream is another option, which may cause some localized skin reaction in a few patients but is easy to use and can be applied by the patient.

Skin preparations should include a pressure sore assessment so that the theatre staff know to take particular precautions to alleviate pressure if the patient is particularly vulnerable.

Identification of right patient and right site

Ms Bailey's identification band should be checked for accuracy. The expected operation and site should be confirmed by the medical staff and the site for operation should be marked on the patient and recorded on the consent form.

Ms Bailey's notes should be collected together with any relevant X-rays or investigation reports and an operation checklist, ready to accompany her to theatre.

Pre-operative prophylactic anti-coagulant, antibiotics

As noted previously, sedatives are not commonly administered pre-operatively, but operations that carry particular risks may require prophylactic antibiotics or anti-coagulants. For example, some orthopaedic operations are associated with prolonged periods of immobility and therefore anti-coagulants may be prescribed to reduce potential blood clotting. Gastro-intestinal or arterial surgery carries a higher risk of post-operative wound infection and therefore a course of antibiotics may be started pre-operatively and given throughout the post-operative period.

Removal and storage of valuables

To prevent loss or damage, all jewellery and hairgrips should be removed and stored in safekeeping. Wedding rings should be taped to prevent burns from diathermy.

Clothing and hygiene

Having washed, Ms Bailey should put on a clean gown and return to a bed made up with clean linen. Ideally, all underwear should be removed and hair may be covered by a disposable cap or tied back depending on local policies. Ms Bailey should be asked to empty her bladder before transfer to theatre to prevent discomfort and possible incontinence during the procedure.

Transfer to theatre

Before transfer to theatre there is usually a checklist to be completed. The following is an example:

- confirm identity by band and verbally
- confirm operation, site and marking
- baseline observations recorded
- time of last food and drink recorded
- whether a pre-med was given; if so what time, and drug details
- presence of any loose teeth, caps or crowns
- dentures removed
- bladder emptied
- whether a hearing aid is used and, if so, is it with the patient for use in recovery?
- removal of glasses or contact lenses
- special skin preparation completed, including hair removal
- jewellery removed or taped
- valuables stored
- cosmetics and clothing removed
- wearing a theatre gown
- consent form completed
- X-rays with patient
- notes with patient
- handover-nurse's signature.

This checklist should be completed before Ms Bailey leaves the ward and confirmed on handover to the theatre nurse. Handover may occur in the anaesthetic room or a special waiting area. The patient may be taken on their bed or walk depending on the planned operation, but should be accompanied by a nurse from the ward.

Evaluation

Was the checklist completed fully? Was Ms Bailey fully prepared for the surgical procedure?

NURSING PROBLEM 12.3

Problem: Ms Bailey needs to be prepared psychologically for the operation and any changes in body image.

Goal: Ms Bailey has her questions answered and her anxieties relieved.

Intervention: psychological preparation for surgery

The pre-operative psychological needs of patients are complex areas for discussion, and cannot be addressed adequately within the confines of this chapter. However, some key aspects for consideration follow below.

Relieving pre-operative anxiety

It has been known for some time that pre-operative information will reduce a patient's anxiety, but it is now acknowledged that not all information is appropriate. It is suggested that preparation should be responsive to the patient's preferred approach to coping with health problems. She may adopt a coping style which is 'vigilant': that is, requiring a large amount of information in order to be fully prepared and aware of every eventuality, thus feeling in full control of the situation. The opposite coping style would be 'avoidant': requiring only the minimum information from health care professionals (Mitchell 2000), as a means of reducing the stress associated with a health problem. Therefore information should be given sensitively depending on the patient's individual needs, and the nurse needs to be alert to communication signals that may indicate that the information has been sufficient, too much or too complex.

Preparation for altered body image

Surgical incisions when healed will leave a scar, but for some operations the impact will be further-reaching than just a physical scar. Patients undergoing operations such as hysterectomy, amputations, breast surgery, or stoma formation, to name but a few, will have to make mental adjustments to their change in appearance, and possibly go through a bereavement process whereby they come to terms with a change in body image. Meeting other patients who have gone through a similar experience or talking to a clinical nurse specialist can help to begin the adjustment process. Preparation for surgery should therefore include consideration of the impact upon a patient's visual appearance or role in the community. For example, a hysterectomy may make a woman feel she has lost her femininity, or a stoma may have implications for a man who follows a manual trade.

Evaluation

Has Ms Bailey made mental adjustments to her condition? Has she received sufficient information for her needs? Does she need additional information or counselling?

Post-operative care

Preparation should be made on the ward to receive a patient on return from theatre:

- Suction and oxygen should be placed beside the bed and checked to ensure they are working.
- IV stands or bed cradles should be placed ready for use.
- The bed space located in a position for ease of observation.
- The bed is prepared with clean linen.

Immediate post-operative care is undertaken in the recovery room by specially trained nurses, who ensure that the patient has fully recovered from anaesthesia, and that her general condition is stable enough to allow transfer to the ward. The time spent in the recovery room may vary from a few hours to several days in high-dependency care, depending on the surgical procedure.

The essential care in the immediate post-operative period consists of:

- maintenance of a clear airway and breathing
- general observation and monitoring of vital signs to detect haemorrhage or deterioration in condition
- relief of pain and discomfort
- monitoring fluid balance.

NURSING PROBLEM 12.4

Problem: Ms Bailey is to be transferred from recovery room to ward following safe recovery from anaesthesia.

Goal: Ms Bailey is safely transferred between departments and is fully awake.

Intervention: handover of a patient from recovery staff

Maintenance of airway, breathing and oxygenation

Ms Bailey should be fully conscious and rousable, although probably a little sleepy, but able to maintain her own airway. She may require oxygen therapy for a time as she is a smoker. Oxygen should be prescribed by the anaesthetist, and recorded in the notes if it is to continue when Ms Bailey returns to the ward. Skin colour should be observed for evidence of cyanosis, and pulse oximetry may be required on return to the ward.

Baseline observations

Observations of temperature, pulse, respirations and blood pressure should be taken to detect early signs of shock, hypoxia or other complications. These observations will become less frequent as Ms Bailey's condition improves, but will need to be closely monitored on her return to the ward. A rise in temperature after a day or so may indicate the development of other complications such as a wound or chest infection.

Fluid balance

Many types of surgery require fluid replacement by IV therapy (IVT), and guidelines for IV care should be followed (see Chapter 7). The IV site should be checked on handover so that the ward nurse is familiar with the current progress of the regime, and the condition of the IV site. Further IV fluids should be prescribed for administration on the ward.

A fluid balance chart may be commenced in recovery or on arrival on the ward, and all oral or intravenous fluids should be noted. Should the patient not require IVT, oral fluids should not be commenced until the patient is fully awake, to reduce potential vomiting and inhalation.

Urine output should be monitored and recorded to ensure that the kidneys are fully functioning following surgery. If a urinary catheter is in place output will be monitored to ensure that fluids administered during surgery are excreted and that the catheter drainage system is patent. If the patient is not catheterized it should be recorded if urine has been passed, and on return to the ward the urine output should continue to be monitored. If urine has not been passed within eight hours of the operation, urine retention may be developing and every effort should be taken to encourage the patient to pass urine (see Chapter 10).

If a nasogastric tube is in place, the drainage and aspirate should be monitored and recorded so that an accurate fluid balance can be maintained.

Nausea and vomiting (PONV)

About 30 per cent of patients who undergo surgery every year will experience PONV, and this number is increased to 40 per cent for gynaecological patients (Jolley 2001). Preventative measures as in pre-operative preparation can reduce PONV. The administration of anti-emetics and monitoring of their effects will help (see Chapter 10).

Pain relief

Pain relief can be by opioids, non-steroidal anti-inflammatory drugs (NSAID) or local anaesthetic (Hutchings 1995). They may be given orally, rectally, by injection, or by PCA. Sufficient pain relief should be administered to enable Ms Bailey to move about in bed as necessary and to rest comfortably. The amount, type and frequency of pain relief should be recorded on the prescription sheet, and the handover should include the time of the last dose. Adequate pain relief speeds recovery and encourages early mobilization, thus reducing potential post-operative complications. As Ms Bailey is a smoker, she must have enough pain relief to enable her to cough and expectorate effectively, but not depress her respiratory rate. A pain assessment chart may be used to monitor effectiveness of the analgesia.

Wound

The wound should be observed in the recovery room for signs of leakage or bleeding. Any wound drainage should be monitored, and if there is leakage through the dressing the wound should have additional dressings placed on top, rather than disturb the incision and interrupt clot formation. The wound dressing should be checked at regular intervals on return to the ward to ensure that there is minimal oozing.

Patients who have drainage bottles or bags should have the quantity and consistency of fluid monitored. Gynaecological patients may have a sanitary towel in place and vaginal discharge and bleeding should be monitored when other post-operative observations are recorded.

If there are any abnormalities in any of these aspects of care, they should be reported to senior staff for reassessment and further intervention.

Evaluation

Has Ms Bailey returned from recovery fully awake and conscious? Is her pain relief effective? Is her fluid balance satisfactory? Is the wound dry and comfortable?

NURSING PROBLEM 12.5

Problem: Ms Bailey needs to recover from surgical intervention with no complications.

Goal: Ms Bailey makes a safe and uncomplicated recovery from surgery.

Intervention: post-operative care

Recommencing fluids and diet

If an operation has included handling of the gastro-intestinal tract then bowel sounds must be confirmed before oral fluids are recommenced, otherwise paralytic ileus may develop and cause the patient unnecessary distress. If the GI tract is not involved and Ms Bailey is not feeling nauseated, small sips of fluid may be commenced two hours post anaesthesia (Jolley 2001). If fluids trigger vomiting, then return to nil by mouth until it resolves.

Once fluids have been tolerated there may be a return to normal diet as soon as Ms Bailey feels able. Additional roughage may need to be included in the diet to prevent constipation occurring, since Ms Bailey will not want to strain to have her bowels open as it may cause discomfort at the incision site.

Pain relief

Pain relief should follow the regime prescribed by the anaesthetist. If inadequate, Ms Bailey will not be able to return to full mobility quickly and therefore will be at risk of developing complications. Oral medication should be prescribed and commenced as intramuscular or intravenous pain relief is reduced.

Mobilization

Early mobilization will promote recovery and early discharge. Again, adequate pain relief is essential in promoting mobilization. When first getting up after an operation, the patient should be encouraged to take it slowly and steadily, as hurrying may cause fainting. Encourage Ms Bailey to change position in bed to relieve pressure points, stimulate her circulation and encourage deep breathing and coughing.

Wound care

The wound should be allowed to heal with minimal intervention. Some studies have suggested that the original wound dressing may be removed after 24–48 hours and a protective film be placed over the wound for protection and patient comfort (Briggs 1997). Local guidelines for wound care should be followed. The wound should be checked for signs of infection.

Discharge plan

This will include consideration of any special needs like wound dressings, stoma care or if a walking aid is required. Special instructions for continuing care at home should be given to the patient in writing. For example, certain exercises may be required to strengthen muscles weakened during surgery. Information as to when driving, lifting, sexual activity or work can be safely resumed will be helpful for Ms Bailey, so that she can plan her recovery time at home.

Evaluation

Has Ms Bailey had an uneventful recovery from surgical intervention? Has she been able to be discharged as planned?

Further reading

Briggs M (1997) Principles of closed surgical wound care. Journal of Wound Care 6(6): 288–92.

Dawson S (2000) Principles of pre-operative preparation. In Manley K, Bellman L (eds), Surgical Nursing: Advancing Practice. Edinburgh: Churchill Livingstone.

Finlay T (1996) Making sense of bowel preparation. Nursing Times 92(45): 38–39.

Hung P (1992) Pre-operative fasting of patients undergoing elective surgery. British Journal of Nursing 1(6): 286–87.

Hutchings P (1995) Advances in anaesthesia: some recent developments in techniques for short stay surgery. British Journal of Theatre Nursing 5(1): 13–15.

Jolley S (2001) Managing post-operative nausea and vomiting. Nursing Standard 15(40): 47–52.

Mitchell M (2000) Nursing intervention for pre-operative anxiety. Nursing Standard 14(37): 40–43.

Seymour S (2000) Pre-operative fluid restrictions: hospital policy and clinical practice. British Journal of Nursing 9(14): 925–30.

Simmons M (1998) Pre-operative skin preparation. Professional Nurse 13(7): 446–47.

Thomas N (1995) Patient-controlled analgesia. Nursing Standard 9(35): 31–35.

Torrance C, Serginson E (1997) Surgical Nursing, 12th edn. London: Bailliere Tindall.

References

Abley C (1997) Teaching elderly patients how to use inhalers: a study to evaluate an education programme on inhaler technique for elderly patients. Journal of Advanced Nursing 25(4): 699–708.

ACHCEW (1997) Hungry in Hospital? London: Association of Community Health Councils of England and Wales.

Addison R (1999) Fluid intake and continence care: practical procedures for nurses. Nursing Times: 37(1): Supp.

Addison R, Ness W, Abulafi M, Swift I (2000) How to administer enemas and suppositories. Nursing Times 96(6; Supplement): 3–4.

Amarigiri SV, Lees TA (1999) Review: graduated compression stockings prevent deep vein thrombosis in patients who are in hospital. Cochrane Data Base Systematic Review 2000(3): CD001484.

Amoore J, Dewar D, Ingram P, Lowe D (2001) Syringe pumps and start up time: ensuring safe practice. Nursing Standard 15(17): 43–45.

AORN (1996) Recommended practices for maintaining a sterile field. AORN Journal 64(5): 817–21.

Arrowsmith H (1996) Nursing management of patients receiving gastrostomy feeding. British Journal of Nursing 2(21): 1053–58.

Arrowsmith H (1997) Malnutrition in hospital: detection and consequences. British Journal of Nursing 6(19): 1131–35.

Atterbury C, Wilkinson J (2000) Blood transfusion. Nursing Standard 14(34): 47–52.

Aucken S, Crawford B (1998) Neurological assessment. In Guerrero D (ed.), Neuro-Oncology for Nurses. London: Whurr.

Ayliffe GAJ, Babb JR, Taylor LJ (1999) Hospital-Acquired Infection: Principles and Prevention, 3rd edn. Oxford: Butterworth-Heinemann.

Baeyens T, Macduff C, West B (2000) Nutritional guidelines for community nurses. Nursing Times Plus 96(8): 4–5.

Baillie L, Arrowsmith V (2001) Meeting elimination needs. In Baillie L (ed.), Developing Practical Nursing Skills. London: Arnold.

Baker F, Smith L, Stead L, Soulsby C (1999) Inserting a nasogastric tube. Nursing Times 95(7): Insert 2p.

Bandolier (1997) Constipation. Bandolier 46 (December): 3. Also http://www.jr2.ox. ac.uk/bandolier/band46/b46-3.html.

Bates B, Hoekelman RA (2000) Guide to Physical Exam and History Taking, 6th edn. On CD-ROM. Philadelphia, PA: Lippincott, Williams and Wilkins.

BCSH (1999) Guidelines for the administration of blood and blood components and the management of the transfused patient. British Committee for Standards in Haematology. Transfusion Medicine 9: 227–38.

Beevers G, Lip GYH, O'Brien E (2001) ABC of hypertension: blood pressure measurement. British Medical Journal 322(7293): 1043–47.

Bell C (1995) Is this what the doctor ordered? Accuracy of oxygen therapy prescribed and delivered in hospital. Professional Nurse 10(5): 297–300.

Beyea SC, Nicholl LH (1995) Administration of medications via the intramuscular route: an integrative review of the literature and research-based protocol for the procedure. Applied Nursing Research 5(1): 23–33.

Black P (2000) Practical stoma care. Nursing Standard 14(41): 47–53.

Bliss DZ, Lehmann S (1999) Tube feeding: administration tips. Registered Nurse 62(8): 29–32.

Bond S (ed.) (1997) Eating Matters. Centre for Health Services Research and The Institute for Health of the Elderly, University of Newcastle.

Bradbury M, Cruickshank JL (2000) Blood transfusion: crucial steps in maintaining safe practice. British Journal of Nursing 9(3): 134–38.

Braun S, Preston P, Smith RN (1998) Getting a better read on thermometry. Registered Nurse 61(3): 57–60.

Bree-Williams FJ, Waterman H (1996) An examination of nurses' practices when performing aseptic technique for wound dressings. Journal of Advanced Nursing 23(1): 48–54.

Briggs M (1997) Principles of closed surgical wound care. Journal of Wound Care 6(6): 288–92.

Briggs M, Wilson S, Fuller A (1996) The principles of aseptic technique in wound care. Professional Nurse 11(12): 805–12.

British National Formulary. London: British Medical Association and British Pharmaceutical Society.

British Society of Gastroenterology (1996) Guidelines on Artificial Nutrition Support. London: British Society of Gastroenterology Publications.

Brown J, Meikle J, Webb C (1991) Collecting midstream specimens for urine – the research base. Nursing Times 87(13): 49–52.

Buckley PM, MacFie J (1997) Enteral nutrition in critically ill patients – a review. Care of the Critically Ill 13(1): 7–10.

Burden M (1994) A practical guide to insulin injections. Nursing Standard 8(29): 25–29.

Burglass EA (1995) Oral hygiene. British Journal of Nursing 4(9): 516–19.

Burnham P (2000) A guide to nasogastric tube insertion. Nursing Times Plus 96(8): 6–7.

Campbell J (1995) Injections. Professional Nurse 10(7): 455–58.

Campbell S (2001) Commentary on review: graduated compression stockings prevent deep vein thrombosis in patients who are in hospital. Evidence-Based Nursing 4: 20.

Carriquiry AL (1999) Assessing the prevalence of nutrient inadequacy. Public Health Nutrition 2(1): 23–33.

References

Clay M (2001) Nutritious, enjoyable food in nursing homes. Nursing Standard 15(19): 47–53.

Cockshott WP et al. (1982) Intramuscular or intralipomatous injections. New England Journal of Medicine 307(6): 356–58.

Colagiovanni L (2000) Preventing and clearing blocked feeding tubes. Nursing Times Plus 96(17): 3–4.

Colleran Cook M (1999) Nurses' six rights for safe medication administration. Massachusetts Nurse 69(6): 8.

Copeman J (1999) Nutritional Care for Older People: A Guide to Good Practice. London: Age Concern.

Cortis JD (1997) Nutrition and the hospitalized patient. British Journal of Nursing 6(12): 666–74.

Covington TP, Trattler MR (1997) Learn how to zero in on the safest site for an IM injection. Nursing (January): 62–63.

Cowan T (1996) Nebulisers for use in the community. Professional Nurse 12(3): 215–20.

Cronin K, Wallois M (2000) Temperature taking in the ICU: which route is best? Australian Critical Care 13(2): 59–64.

Dawson S (2000) Principles of pre-operative preparation. In Manley K, Bellman L (eds), Surgical Nursing: Advancing Practice. Edinburgh: Churchill Livingstone.

Department of Health (2001a) Standard principles for preventing hospital-acquired infections. Journal of Hospital Infection 47: S21–S37. See also http://www.idealibrary.com.

Department of Health (2001b) Guidelines for preventing infections associated with the insertion and maintenance of short-term indwelling urethral catheters in acute care. Journal of Hospital Infection 47, Supplement S39–46.

Dodd M (1996) Nebuliser therapy: what nurses and patients need to know. Nursing Standard 10(31): 39–42.

Dougherty L (1996) Peripheral venous cannulation – the patient's perspective. Background paper: Clinical Guidelines Workshop. London: Royal College of Physicians Research Unit Publications.

Driscoll A (2000) Managing post-discharge care at home: an analysis of patients' and their carers' perceptions of information received during their stay in hospital. Journal of Advanced Nursing 31(5): 1165–73.

Dunn L, Chrisholm H (1998) Oxygen therapy. Nursing Standard 13(7): 57–64.

Edington J, Kon P, Martyn C (1996) Prevalence of malnutrition in patients in general practice. Clinical Nutrition 15: 60–63.

Edwards SL (2000) Fluid overload and monitoring indices. Professional Nurse 15(9): 568–72.

Evans G (2001) A rationale for oral care. Nursing Standard 15(43): 33–36.

Fell H, Boehm M (1998) Easing the discomfort of oxygen therapy. Nursing Times 94(38): 56–58.

Finkelstein L (1996) Sputum testing for TB: getting good specimens. American Journal of Nursing 96(2): 14.

Finlay T (1996) Making sense of bowel preparation. Nursing Times 92(45): 38–39.

Frawley P (1990) Neurological observations. Nursing Times 86(35): 29–32.

Getliffe K, Dolman M (1997) Promoting Continence: a Clinical and Research Resource. London: Bailliere Tindall.

Glover G, Powell F (1996) Blood transfusion. Continuing Education Article 344. Nursing Standard 10(21): 49–56.

Gould D (2001) Pressure ulcer risk assessment. Primary Health Care 11(5): 43–49.

Grap MJ (1998) Protocols for practice: applying research at the bedside – pulse oximetry. Critical Care Nurse 18(1): 94–99.

Gray A, Murphy M (1999) Guidelines for administering blood and blood components. Nursing Standard 14(13–15): 36–39.

Guenter P, Jones S, Ericson M (1997) Enteral nutrition therapy. Nursing Clinics of North America 32(4): 651–68.

Guillebaud J (2000) Contraception Today, 4th edn. London: Martin Dunitz Ltd.

Hall J (1996) Evaluating asthma patient inhaler technique. Professional Nurse 11(11): 725–29.

Hand H (2001) The use of intravenous therapy. Nursing Standard 15(43): 47–52.

Hecker J (1988) Improved technique in IV therapy. Nursing Times 84(34): 28–33.

Heywood Jones I (1995) Administration of Enemas. Skills Update Book 4. London: Macmillan Magazines Ltd.

Hollingworth H, Kingston JE (1998) Using a non-sterile technique in wound care. Professional Nurse 13(4): 226–29.

Hung P (1992) Pre-operative fasting of patients undergoing elective surgery. British Journal of Nursing 1(6): 286–87.

Hutchings P (1995) Advances in anaesthesia: some recent developments in techniques for short stay surgery. British Journal of Theatre Nursing 5(1): 13–15.

Infection Control Nurses Association (1997) Guidelines for Hand Hygiene. ICNA.

Iyer PW, Camp HN (1999) Nursing Documentation: A Nursing Process Approach, 3rd edn. St Louis: Mosby Inc.

Jain P, Kavuru MS, Emerman CL, Ahmad M (1998) Utility of peak expiratory flow monitoring. Chest: The Cardiopulmonary Journal 114(3): 861–76.

Jennett B, Teasdale G (1974) Assessment of coma and impaired consciousness. Lancet 2: 81–84.

Jevon P, Ewens B (2001) Assessment of a breathless patient. Nursing Standard 15(16): 48–53.

Jolley S (2001) Managing post-operative nausea and vomiting. Nursing Standard 15(40): 47–52.

Kamm MA, Lennard Jones JE (1994) Constipation. Petersfield: Wrightson Biomedical Publishing Ltd.

Katsma D, Smith G (1997) Analysis of needle path during intramuscular injection. Nursing Research 46(5): 288–92.

Kennedy JF (1997) Enteral feeding for the critically ill patient. Nursing Standard 11(33): 39–43.

Lamb J (1996) Potential problems with the administration of drugs through venous lines. Background paper: Clinical Guidelines Workshop. London: Royal College of Physicians Research Unit Publications.

Ledger D (2000) Ensuring that your patient eats enough. Nursing Times 96(8; NT Plus): 2.

Leech K, McDonnell J (1999) Food, Fluids and Fibre. Colchester: New Possibilities NHS Trust.

Lifecare (2000) Product Information. Market Harborough: Lifecare Hospital Supplies.

References

Lindsay R (1998) Management of Postmenopausal Health: Where Are We Now? Proceedings of a Satellite Symposium at the 6th Bath Conference on Osteoporosis. Reed Healthcare Publishing.

Loan T, Magnuson B, Williams S (1998) Debunking six myths about enteral feeding. Nursing 28(8): 43–9.

Long BC, Phipps WJ, Cassmeyer VL (1995) Adult Nursing: a Nursing Process Approach. London: Mosby.

Lord LM (1997) Enteral access devices. Nursing Clinics of North America 32(4): 685–704.

Lowry M (1998) Trauma, emergency nursing and the Glasgow Coma Scale. Accident and Emergency Nursing 6(3): 143–48.

McConnell EA (1998) Clinical do's and don't's: giving medications through an enteral feeding device. Nursing 28(3): 66.

McConnell EA (1999) Clinical do's and don't's: performing pulse oximetry. Nursing 29(11): 17.

Manley K, Bellman L (eds) (2000) Surgical Nursing: Advancing Practice. Edinburgh: Churchill Livingstone.

Manolio TA, Weinmann GG, Buist AS, Furberg CD, Pinsky JL, Hurd SH (1997) Pulmonary function testing in population-based studies. American Journal of Respiratory and Critical Care Medicine 156(3, Pt.1): 1004–10.

Masoorli S (1995) Infusion therapy lawsuits: an occupational hazard. Journal of Intravenous Nursing 18(2): 88–91.

Mathews PJ (1997) Using a peak flow meter: monitoring the air waves. Nursing 27(6): 57–59.

May D (2001) Infection Control: Understanding the Basic Concepts. Nursing Standard Essential Guide. Harrow: RCN.

Mayor S (2000) Hospital-acquired infections kill 5000 patients a year in England. British Medical Journal 321: 1370.

Medical Devices Agency (1995) Device Bulletin Infusion Systems. May DB 9503.

Metcalf C (1999) Stoma care: empowering patients through teaching practical skills. British Journal of Nursing 8(9): 593–600.

Metheny NM (1990) Why worry about IV fluids? American Journal of Nursing 90(6): 50–55.

Millam D (1988) Managing complications of IV therapy. Nursing 18(3): 34–43.

Milligan F (1999) Male sexuality and catheterization: a review of the literature. Nursing Standard 13(38): 43–47.

Mitchell M (2000) Nursing intervention for pre-operative anxiety. Nursing Standard 14(37): 40–43.

Moore J (1995) Assessment of nurse-administered hygiene. Nursing Times 91(9): 40–41.

Morling S (1998) Infusion devices: risks and user responsibilities. British Journal of Nursing 7(1): 13–19.

Morrison C (2000) Helping patients to maintain a healthy fluid balance. NT Plus: Nursing Times 96(31): 3–4.

Muers M, Corris P (1997) Current best practice for nebuliser treatment. Thorax: the Journal of the British Thoracic Society 52(Supp. 2).

Naysmith MR, Nicholson J (1998) Nasogastric drug administration. Professional Nurse 13(7): 424–27.

Nettina SM (2000) The Lippincott Manual of Nursing Practice, 6th edn. On CD-ROM. Philadelphia, PA: Lippincott, Williams and Wilkins.

NHS Centre for Reviews and Dissemination (1995) The Prevention and Treatment of Pressure Sores. York: NHS CRD.

NHS Direct Online (2001) http://www.healthcareguide.nhsdirect.nhs.uk/conditions/lice/lice.stm (accessed 26/09/01).

Nicol M, Bavin C, Bedford-Turner S, Cronin P, Rawlings-Anderson K (2000) Essential Nursing Skills. Edinburgh: Mosby.

Noble JG, Menzies J, Cox PJ, Edwards L (1990) Midnight removal: an improved approach of catheter removal. British Journal of Urology 65(6): 615–17.

O'Brien E, Fitzgerald D (1991) The history of indirect blood pressure measurement. In O'Brien E, O'Malley K (eds), Blood Pressure Measurement: Handbook of Hypertension. Amsterdam: Elsevier.

O'Callaghan C, Barry P (1997) Spacer devices in the treatment of asthma. British Medical Journal 314(7087): 1061–62.

O'Shea J (1999) Factors contributing to medication errors: a literature review. Journal of Clinical Nursing 8(5): 496–504.

Oliver L (1997) Wound cleansing. Nursing Standard 11(20): 47–51.

Owen A (1998) Respiratory assessment revisited. Nursing 28(4): 48–49.

Parker L (1999) IV devices and related infections: causes and complications. British Journal of Nursing 8(22): 1491–98.

Pearson AB, Vaughan M, Fitzgerald (1996) Nursing Models for Practice, 2nd edn. Oxford: Butterworth-Heinemann.

Pedley G (1999) Maintaining healthy skin. In Redfern S, Ross F (eds), Nursing Older People. London: Churchill Livingstone.

Penzer R, Finch M (2001) Promoting healthy skin on older people. Nursing Standard 15(34): 46–52.

Peragallo-Dittko V (1997) Rethinking subcutaneous injection technique. American Journal of Nursing 97(5): 71–72.

Perry AG, Potter PA (1998) Pocket Guide to Basic Skills and Procedures, 4th edn. St Louis: Mosby.

Perry L (1997) Nutrition: a hard nut to crack. An exploration of the knowledge, attitudes and activities of qualified nurses in relation to nutritional nursing care. Journal of Clinical Nursing 6(4): 315–24.

Pickstone M (ed.) (1999) A Pocketbook for Safer IV Therapy. Kent: Scitech Educational Ltd.

Potter PA, Perry AG (eds) (1997) Fundamentals of Nursing: Concepts, Process and Practice, 4th edn. St Louis: Mosby.

Proehl JA (1992) The Glasgow Coma Scale: do it and do it right. Journal of Emergency Nursing 18(5): 421–23.

RCN (1996) RCN Statement on Feeding and Nutrition in Hospitals. London: RCN.

RCN (1997) Universal Precautions. London: RCN.

RCN (1999) Royal College of Nursing Guidance for Nurses Giving Intravenous Therapy. London: RCN.

Reilly H (1998) Enteral feeding: an overview of indications and techniques. British Journal of Nursing 7(8): 461–67.

Rodger MA, King L (2000) Drawing up and administering intramuscular injections: a review of the literature. Journal of Advanced Nursing 31(3): 574–82.

Rollins H (1997) A nose for trouble. Nursing Times 93(49): 66–67.

Roper N, Logan W, Tierney A (eds) (1998) The Elements of Nursing: a Model for Nursing Based on a Model of Living. Edinburgh: Churchill Livingstone.

Salter M (ed.) (1988) Altered Body Image: the Nurse's Role. London: Wiley.

Sander R (1999) Promoting urinary continence in residential care. Nursing Standard 14(13–15): 49–53.

Severine JE, McKenzie N (1997) Advances in temperature monitoring: a far cry from 'shake and take'. Nursing 27(5 Suppl.): 1–10.

Seymour S (2000) Pre-operative fluid restrictions: hospital policy and clinical practice. British Journal of Nursing 9(14): 925–30.

Shah S (1999) Neurological assessment. Nursing Standard 13(22): 49–54.

SHOT (1999) Serious Hazards of Transfusion Annual Report 1997–1998. Manchester: SHOT.

Simmonds BP (1983) CDC guidelines for the prevention and control of nosocomial infections: guidelines for the prevention of intravascular infections. American Journal of Infection Control 11(5): 183–89.

Simmons M (1998) Pre-operative skin preparation. Professional Nurse 13(7): 446–47.

Simpson L (2001) Indwelling urethral catheters: reducing the risk of potential complications through proactive management. Primary Health Care 11(2): 57–64.

Spencer RC (1996) Epidemiology of venous lines. Background paper: Clinical Guidelines Workshop. London: Royal College of Physicians Research Unit Publications.

Springhouse (2000) Nurse's Clinical Guide: Medication Administration. Springhouse, PA: Springhouse Corporation.

Springhouse (2000) Nursing Procedures, 3rd edn. Springhouse, PA: Springhouse Corporation.

Springhouse (2002) Assessment Made Incredibly Easy, 2nd edn. Springhouse, PA: Springhouse Publishing Company.

Stavem K, Saxholm H, Erikssen J (2000) Tympanic or rectal temperature measurement? A cost minimization analysis. Scandinavian Journal of Infectious Diseases 32(3): 299–301.

Talbot L, Curtis L (1996) The challenges of assessing skin indicators in people of color. Home Healthcare Nurse 14(3): 167–73.

Thomas N (1995) Patient-controlled analgesia. Nursing Standard 9(35): 31–35.

Thomas S (2000) New continence guidance. Primary Health Care 10(6): 20–21.

Thomson I (1998) Teaching the skills to cope with a stoma. Nursing Times 94(4): 55–56.

Tierney A, Worth A, King C, Macmillan M (1994) Older patients' experiences of discharge from hospital. Nursing Times 90(21): 36–39.

Togshill PJ (1997) Essential Medical Practice. London: Arnold.

Tomlinson D (1987) To clean or not to clean. Nursing Times (March 4): 71–75.

Torrance C, Semple MC (1998) Recording temperature. Nursing Times 94(2): Practical Procedures for Nurses Supplement.

Torrance C, Serginson E (1997) Surgical Nursing, 12th edn. London: Bailliere Tindall.

Turner G (1996) Oral care. Nursing Standard 10(28): 51–54.

UK Health Departments (1998) Guidance for Clinical Healthcare Workers: Protection Against Blood-borne Viruses. Recommendations of the Expert Advisory group on AIDS and the Advisory Group on Hepatitis: http:/www.open.gov.uk/doh/chcguidl.htm.

UKCC (1992) Code of Conduct. London: UKCC.

UKCC (1998) Guidelines for Records and Record Keeping. London: UKCC.

UKCC (2000) Guidelines for the Administration of Medications. London: UKCC.

UKCC (2001) Disguising medication. Register (Autumn) 37: 7.

Ward J, Rollins H (1999) Screening for malnutrition. Nursing Standard 14(8): 49–53.

Watson R (1998) Controlling body temperature in adults. Nursing Standard 12(20): 49–55.

White G (1998) Nutritional supplements and tube feeds: what is available? British Journal of Nursing 7(5): 246, 248–50.

White S (2000) A multidisciplinary PEG service and the nurse specialist. Nursing Times Plus 96(49): 6–9.

Whitson M (1996) Intravenous therapy in the older adult, special needs and considerations. Journal of Intravenous Nursing 19(5): 251–55.

Wilkinson R (1996) Nurses' concerns about IV therapy and devices. Nursing Standard 10(35): 35–37.

Williams A (1996) How to avoid mistakes in medicine administration. Nursing Times 92(13): 40–41.

Wilson J (1995) Infection Control in Clinical Practice. London: Bailliere Tindall.

Wilson J (1997) Control and prevention of infection in catheter care. Nurse Prescriber/Community Nurse 3(5): 39–40.

Wilson J, Arnold C, Connor R, Cusson R (1996) Evaluation of oxygen delivery with the use of nasopharyngeal catheters and nasal cannulas. Neonatal Network: Journal of Neonatal Nursing 15(4): 15–22.

Woodrow P (1999) Pulse oximetry. Nursing Standard 13(42): 42–47.

Woollon S (1997) Selection of intravenous and infusion pumps. Professional Nurse Supplement 12(8): S14–S15.

Workman BA (1999) Peripheral intravenous therapy management. Nursing Standard 14(4): 53–60.

Workman BA (1999) Safe injection techniques. Nursing Standard 13(39): 47–53.

Xavier G (1999) Asepsis. Nursing Standard 13(36): 49–53.

Index

manometer 25–6
manual dexterity 7, 13, 201, 215, 217–18
incontinence 237–8, 242
manual handling 87, 253–4, 256
mastectomy 24
meatal area 241, 245–6, 301, 303–4
mechanical pumps 151, 154–5, 156–7, 166
medication 21, 36, 93–133, 191, 226, 233
assessment 4, 12, 14
calculating doses 93, 95, 99–100, 102, 310
compatibility with lignocaine 302
decubitus ulcers 86–7
elimination 235, 238, 262–3, 265
infection control 48, 53
nausea and vomiting 273
pre-operative care 310–11, 315
respiratory care 179, 191, 196
see also drug administration
Medicines Act (1968) 93
melaena 237
menstruation 7, 257
mercury thermometers 28–33
metered dose inhalers (MDIs) 200, 201–3, 206
Methicillin-resistant Staphylococcus aureus (MRSA) 48–9, 53–4, 57, 277
microscopy, culture and sensitivity (MC&S) 193, 232, 240–1
IVT 163, 164
urinary catheters 305
wound swabs 294, 296–7
micturition *see* urine and urination
minerals and nutrition 215
Mini-Wright peak flow meter 185
Misuse of Drugs Act (1971) 93, 109
Misuse of Drugs Regulations (1985) 93
mobility 13, 78–9, 87, 321
assessment 7, 13, 15
complications of bed-rest 78–80, 83–8
constipation 261, 263
elimination 235, 237–8, 252, 257, 261, 263

personal hygiene 60, 61–2, 65, 71, 76
post-operative care 320, 321
mood 4, 6, 15
motor response and consciousness 34–5, 38–41
mouth and oral care 28–30, 71–4, 101–5, 193, 229
drug administration 93, 101–5, 107, 115, 123, 125, 127, 319
fluid balance 134–5, 136–8, 140–1, 142
nutrition 216–17
personal hygiene 60, 62, 71–4
temperature 19, 27, 28–20, 31
mucous membrane 183, 188, 208, 276
infection control 49, 50
multiple sclerosis 14

nails and nail beds 39, 65, 183, 312, 313
nasogastric (NG) tubes 106–11, 214, 220–9
compared with PEG tubes 229–30, 233
drug administration 105, 106–11
feeding 106–7, 109, 214, 220–9
fluid balance 135, 139
kinking 108
nausea and vomiting 274
post-operative care 319
nasopharyngeal suctioning 178, 207–8, 209–11
nausea 104, 235, 272–4, 311–12
fluid balance 137
IVT 164
PEG tubes 232
post-operative care 319, 321
nebulizers 178, 191, 196–8
needle-phobic patients 120, 145
needlestick injuries 47, 50, 116, 123
neonates 54, 154
neoplasms 264
nerve injury 161, 163–4
neurological dysfunction 14, 236, 238, 263
observations 20, 38, 41
new variant CJD 170